HIGHWAY HYPODERMICS:

TRAVEL NURSING 2017

By

Epstein LaRue, RN, CGM
(Certified Grad-level Management)

With contributing authors,
Joseph Smith, RRT, EA
Aaron Highfill, RN, CFRN

Highway Hypodermics:
Travel Nursing 2017

Trade Paperback ISBN: 978-1-935188-81-0
Ebook ISBN: 978-1-935188-82-7

Edited by Star Publish LLC
Interior Design by: Star Publish LLC
Cover Design by Epstein LaRue

Published in 2016 by Star Publish, LLC

Printed in the United States of America

A Star Publish Book
www.starpublishllc.com
Pennsylvania, U.S.A.

Dedicated to:

Those travel companies who have supported highwayhypodermics.com for the last 10 years!

Freedom Healthcare
www.freedomhcs.com

TaleMed
www.talemed.com

IPI Travel
www.ipitravel.com

Millenia Medical Staffing
www.milleniamedical.com

INTERIOR CONTENTS:

Chapter One

An Introduction To Travel Nursing

"All that wander, are not lost."
(JRR Tolkien)

In 2003 I entered the exciting world of travel nursing. Since that time, I have crisscrossed the United States three different times, experienced the Grand Canyon, whirled my way through Hurricane Wilma, and made several trips to visit our neighbors in Canada. During the last 10 years, not only have I changed as a nurse and traveler, but I have seen plenty travel nursing companies exceed in the business while many have succumbed to their injuries.

At the time of writing this, the five largest travel companies are: AMN Healthcare (American Mobile, Medical Express, Nurse Choice), Cross Country Healthcare (Cross Country TravCorp, Nova Pro, CRU48), Medical Solutions, CHG Healthcare Services (RN Network), and Aureus Medical Group. The top five smaller companies include: Health Providers Choice, Talemed, Premier Healthcare Professionals, IPI Travel, and OneStaff Medical.

In 2013 I did my first search of specialties and found the Med/Surg/Tele, ICU, and ER had the most jobs. This year, I found that the top specialties are MS (3794), ICU (3061), OR (2414), ER (2118), Tele (1906), OB (1588), and PICU/NICU (1108) for a total of 15,989 jobs. Medical/Surgical still holds the lead, even after splitting Telemetry needs out. In 2013, ICU counted 2583 jobs while ER counted 1764 jobs, this year we found that ICU had 3061 jobs and ER had 2118 jobs, which both represent a 20% increase. (Travel Nursing Jobs, 2016).

One of the biggest staffing questions is the use of agency and/or travel staff. In a recent healthcare staffing study presented by KMPG, it was reported that once you look at the total cost of training a new nurse (orientation, benefits, and continuing education) it is cost effective to hire agency or travel nurses to fill those spots. The great thing about travel nurses is that we are experienced nurses that are trained to hit the floor running (Institute, 2011).

The big world of travel nursing and allied health is exciting, but it can also be very stressful. You need to educate yourself in the way of the travel healthcare world so that you can navigate the high seas with open eyes. That has been my purpose for the last 13 years: to educate nurses and therapist on the field of travel nursing and healthcare through my books, website, and blogs.

What Makes Kay "Epstein LaRue" Slane the Expert?

My life as a nurse started out in 1992 with a graduation to travel nursing in 2003. My only regret then was that I didn't start sooner! But, I always thought that I couldn't go on the road and travel related to the fact that I needed to give my son a "stable" environment. Well, that's a bunch of BS! He learned a lot more on the road and remembers it!

At this time, I had written the novels "*Love At First Type*" about how two people had come together online, and "*Crazy Thoughts of Passion*," my attempt to bring my writing romance world into my nursing world. Those first books were published under the pen name of "Epstein LaRue;" therefore, I continued the tradition when I wrote my first travel nursing books. Eight books later, I can't hide under a pen name, people were catching on that Kay Slane was actually the author, Epstein LaRue. Many times in hospital orientation, people would ask, "Aren't you the gal who writes those travel nursing books?"

When I started investigating the life of a traveling nurse, I wrote everything down and began to make notes about how to find an assignment and where to go. I was frustrated at having to go to multiple website to look up this information and there was only one book out there on traveling nursing, "*Hitting The Road*" by Shalon Weddington.

There ought to be a better way to do things! Soon I had compiled all the information that I had collected into the Highway Hypodermics website. After that I put all that information into a non-fictional work named, "*Highway Hypodermics: Your Road Map To Travel Nursing.*" This book was published in January of 2005 and did okay in sales but things would look brighter!

In January 2007, Star Publish and I put out the second edition, *Highway Hypodermics: Travel Nursing 2007*. In that edition there was a lot of information added about the PBDS test, The Joint Commission, homeschooling and traveling with family. It went to number one on Amazon three times in the nursing trends, issues, and roles category.

In 2009 the third edition of *Highway Hypodermics*, which had the subtitle of "*On The Road Again*" was published, which added the aspects of traveling as an LPN/LVN, Allied Health traveling, and travel nursing when you are coming from other countries. By this time three other books had been written on the travel nursing subject. Two of the three along with my book were all turned into the 2009 USA Book News' annual contest. *Highway Hypodermics: On the Road Again* was a winner that year while the others were finalists!

The fourth edition: *Highway Hypodermics: Travel Nursing 2012* saw even more changes to include: "Traveling With Pets," "the BKAT," "General Testing That is Required," and "The National Association of Travel Healthcare Organizations (NATHO)." All of the nursing stories were new and the travel company profiles have been updated, including several new companies.

In 2015, the fifth edition, most of the chapters were completely rewritten and the format changed just a skosh. Although not all the chapters have been changed, the book has had a total facelift from 10 years ago with chapters reorganized for a better flow. Added to that year's information includes a chapter dedicated to contracts and one solely dedicated to finding the right recruiter. In that book we also concentrated on the traits of a quality travel nurse and how you need to behave once you are on assignment. Travel nurses are one of the biggest stereotyped groups out there. One nurse can ruin your assignment before you even enter the hospital doors.

In 2017, all the chapters have been thoroughly reviewed and updated. I have also enlisted the help of Joseph Smith, RT, Travel Tax, to author the tax chapter, and Aaron Highfill, RN, Flight Nurse, to author the chapter on International Travel. As with the 2015 version, which was released at the 2014 Travelers Conference, this version will also have a release date to correspond to the Travelers Conference, where you can get signatures from all of the Authors.

Not only am I the author of this book series, but I have several Facebook groups for newbie travel nurses, homeschoolers, and healthcare professionals who travel in an RV. I take pride in providing as much time as possible helping traveling healthcare professionals find the best assignments, agencies, and recruiters for their needs.

Why Nursing to Begin With?

Why would someone want to go into a profession where you are begged to work overtime so you can hear from the families a confirmation of the fact that nurses don't have time to take care of patients the way they should. Families are, however, somewhat more tolerant of it because they know that "all hospitals are short-staffed."

Why would you want to run around "like a chicken with its head cut off" for eight hours before you get time to stop long enough to get a drink, go to the restroom, and grab a sandwich on your way back because we can't waste time for lunch? That abscess has to be drained!

Why would someone want to get into a profession where your feet are abused by all the long hours spent traipsing down the corridors of illness? If you are not one of the lucky ones to marry a foot masseur, you'd better learn self-massage techniques and get some comfortable shoes.

Why would anyone want to spend time wiping butts, giving enemas, taking blood, then giving some back, cleaning up vomit, and my personal favorite—cleaning up that stringy sputum!

I am expected to work long hours, contend with ridiculous staffing circumstances, be treated like a dog by the administration, be yelled at by the physicians while dodging the clipboard, and be ridiculed by my nursing colleagues because I am definitely not working as hard as they are and I am not as good as they are.

I never could understand the old saying, "Nurses always eat their young," but that is exactly what we do. The new graduates are inexperienced and "stupid" because they haven't been around the block like we have, but I drag myself out of bed at 4:00 a.m. every morning because I care about the patients I take care of. I don't know why anybody wouldn't want to live the dream of being a nurse!

Career nurses are nurses because we are dedicated to our profession—because we really are concerned about patient care and the health of others. It is just hard to convey to someone else that this profession really does have its high points. If only they could see the patient's son who gives us a hug because we took care of his mother so well as she slipped from this life to the next. If only they could visit with the patient who went into ventricular fibrillation before my eyes and told me "thank you" ten minutes after I had defibrillated her. Making a difference in someone else's life—*that,* my friend, is what nursing is all about.

Another concern for professional nurses is the issue of mandatory overtime. My colleague Melissa James stated, "After working a twelve-hour day shift at the nursing home, the night shift nurse called in. I was then informed by the director of nursing that I would stay or be turned into the state for patient abandonment."

Once being coerced into working those extra shifts, the nurses recognize in their hearts that they should not be touching syringes, handing out medications, or providing medical treatment, but they carry on as instructed because they have a family to feed at home and a nursing license to protect.

Investigative reports show that insomnia has some bearing on more than just a few aspects of nursing implementation, leading to sluggish responses, delayed reaction times, failure to make a start when appropriate, erroneous functions, decelerated thoughts, and a diminished recollection of nursing actions already performed.

Another factor influencing the nursing shortage is the increase of government interventions. With the rules and regulations of Medicare, medical treatment is ruled by money, not by patient need. This also is a factor with insurance entities, including HMOs, PPOs, and private insurance.

The patient's length of stay is governed by the patient's DRG (Diagnostic Related Group). If you have a hernia surgery, the government, not the physicians, tells you when your time is up. As a nurse this bothers me terribly because I see repeat patients that should have been taken care of longer the first time, who have been discharged only to return two weeks later with a severe infection and wound dehiscence. Now we have the new government mandated insurance "Obamacare" that brings a whole new degree of difficulty to the government involvement in healthcare.

Who wants to work with people who have new diseases like vancomycin resistance enterococci (VRE), methicillin resistance staphylococcus aureus (MRSA), AIDS, HIV, tuberculosis, hepatitis, and other life-threatening contagious diseases?

Travel Nursing Basics

Travel nursing is for those nurses who are competent, can hit the floor running, and who have at least two years of experience. The job description also includes working 13 weeks at a hospital, long-term care facility, or home health setting to help out when there are nursing shortages.

You will have many housing options including a fully furnished one-bedroom apartment, corporate housing, an extended stay, or just a plain ole motel room. More and more nurses are finding that it is much easier to take to the road in an RV!

In most situations you will take your own vehicle, but there are some assignments, like Hawaii or Alaska, where the company will provide a rental car or a rental car stipend. You can take your car to Alaska, but it is a long trip! Upon submission to Ketchikan, Alaska, my husband and I also explored taking the ferry from Washington State to Ketchikan. With Hawaii your most sensible option is to fly, although I guess you could take a boat. Some people have their car shipped over there, but more tend to get a rental car or take public transportation. (It's reported that one hospital in Honolulu charges $20 a day just for parking!)

The three major players in the travel nursing field are the hospital, the agency, and the nurse. Hospitals all around the country are having trouble filling all their full time spots with nurses in their general area. When the shortage gets extreme, they put in an "order" for a nurse. These orders specify exactly what they are looking for. For example they would want a nurse who has BLS, ACLS, PALS, and TNCC to work in the ER. They will want BLS and ACLS for the ICU. If you are critical care certified (CCRN), your profile will jump up the manager large pile of profiles on their desk. Usually a hospital will add what they need to a job database, also known as a vendor management system, which we will talk about more later!

Who are looking at the job databases? Travel nursing companies! These companies are compromised usually of a President/CEO, Nursing Manager, Recruiting Manager, and recruiters. If large enough, they will also have a housing and credentialing department. The one that you will have the most contact with is the recruiter! It is his or her job to look at the database to see if there is a hospital that needs you! They look at their list of needs to see if there is a job that fits your experience and certifications.

You, the traveling nurse or therapist, have the biggest job in weeding through all the travel companies to find the perfect assignment at the perfect time. The Internet has made this process easier. I couldn't imagine doing this before the Internet was available, but I know that some did it! Now your job is even easier considering that several websites, including www.highwayhypodermics.com, have travel companies reviews. Highway Hypodermics is also the only website that lists the benefits each company provides. After finding an assignment you like with a company that fits your needs, the travel nurse's profile will be sent to the hospital and hopefully an interview is soon to follow.

After the travel assignment is accepted, the finer details of housing and travel are then worked out. It is your job as a travel nurse to be adaptable and flexible, but on the other hand, don't let them break you! Number one when you get your contract - READ IT CAREFULLY! It's like nursing documentation, if it isn't documented it isn't done! When you get to your assignment remember that you are representing all traveling nurses. If you look bad it has a direct reflection on the travel nursing field. Your job is to go to the hospital, do what they do, and provide quality nursing care.

To help you decide if travel nursing is right for you and to get you started in travel nursing, I urge you to get in the know by downloading our Travel Nursing Newbies Workbook at: http://highwayhypodermics.com/wp/email-sign-up/. By signing up for our newsletter, you will get emails only when we have something major going on, such as a new book, workbook, or website.

Educational Factors

There are travel nursing jobs for all levels of nursing, Certified Nursing Assistants (CNAs), Licensed Practical Nurses (LPN), associate level Registered Nurses (RNs), along with Bachelor prepared RNs, and Master's prepared RNs.

CNAs and LPNs have a harder time finding assignments, but they are out there. I found it easier for these two categories to go with a larger company who has more job openings for these levels. RNs are the most widely sought after nurses. Associate level RNs have absolutely no problems finding jobs in a lot of hospitals, but the larger teaching hospitals and those hospitals with "Magnet" status are starting to require that all RNs have a Bachelor's Degree in Nursing.

The one job level that is becoming more prevalent is traveling nursing managers and supervisors. For this level, it helps to have a Master's in Nursing or at least some Grad-Level classes. Since my Bachelor is in Secondary Science Education, I found a program through Excelsior College in which they are now awarding a Certificate in Graduate-level Nursing Management (CGM). This requires you to take the 4 graduate-level classes and prepares you to take the test to become a Certified Nursing Manager and Leader (CNM-L), which was developed in partnership with the American Association of Critical Care Nurses (AACN).

Certificates are also a great way to get your resume to the top of the resume pile. Other AACN certification programs include Critical Care, Progressive Care, Cardiac Medicine, and Acute Care Nurse Practitioners. Again, the advanced degrees are not required but can help you get to the top of the resume pile.

Why Travel Nursing?

The number one reason that nurses start traveling is for the excellent wages. If you live in the south or a low-paying state and go to the coastal areas, you have the potential to double your take home pay. Yes, your expenses do increase with housing and weekend getaways, but the savings potential is astronomical when compared to working at a lower wage state.

The number two reason nurses travel is to stay out of the politics. One of my colleagues was fed up with being a unit manager. Being in middle management was stressing her out to the max. She left her management position for the open road and hasn't ever looked back. Another friend of mine states that she was tired of all the "riff-raff" that the hospital required. She just wants to go to work, take care of her patients, and then come home.

What really happens is that we trade hospital politics for company politics. This is most especially true if you change companies every 13 to 26 weeks. There are all kinds of credentialing that we have to go through before we can even be considered for an assignment.

Some people travel related to the higher wages. The wage differences between staff and travel used to be a wide margin, but recently this margin has become less and less although staff nurses still think that we are out there making quite a bit more. When you consider the fact that we have a permanent home also with double the expenses, the traveler is making some more but not as much as staff members think we are making. This margin is bigger, though, if you are from a southern state and traveling to the coastal states.

Another great aspect of travel nursing is exploring the country. On our days off you can find us hiking or biking in the great outdoors, shopping at quaint little local shops, or just exploring your new territory. Even if you have only an 8 week assignment, and working every other weekend, you can still sneak in a west weekend, east weekend, north weekend, and south weekend.

Professional growth is another great reason to start travel nursing. There are new technologies entering the medical field all the time. In a smaller hospital you may not see some of the bigger technologies, but you will obtain the knowledge about many different technologies. In a bigger hospital, you can learn all about the higher level of technology. For instance, I have done a lot of smaller critical access facilities; therefore, I know a little bit about everything from fetal monitoring, to cardiac monitoring, to emergency nursing, and rehabilitation. I'm now traveling at a larger hospital, and I was totally amazed the other day when in the middle of a code we got out the ultrasound machine and we knew exactly what was going on with that patient's heart because we could see it!

The one consistent thing I find with travel nursing is that you either love it or hate it. There aren't very many people who are stuck in the middle. For many of us travelers the top question is, "Why didn't I become a traveler sooner?"

Travel Nursing Goals

The diversity of goals is just as broad as the reasons we decided to become nurses to begin with! Many have the goal of traveling through or working in all 50 states and seeing all the National Parks and Monuments.

One of my first goals was to travel the entire distance of the Pacific Coast Highway all the way from San Diego to the Washington state peninsula. We did this in many trips. During one outing, we took the I-5 freeway down to San Diego and then made the trip back up on the Pacific Coast Highway (PCH1). On two other trips we made the journey to San Francisco and up to as far as Garberville, CA. During this time we got to see plenty of lighthouses and enjoyed many state and national parks. While on assignment in Tillamook, Oregon, we made the rest of the journey, from Tillamook down to Garberville, CA, and then on another weekend we went north from Tillamook and followed the coast around the Washington Peninsula through Port Angeles, over to Seattle, WA, down to Portland, OR, and back to Tillamook.

Have fun with your GPS! I was on assignment in the Monterey, CA, area, and one weekend we took off and went south from Monterey to Los Angeles. For the adventure of it all, we set the GPS on "shortest route" to Big Sur, and it took us OVER the mountain.

I put this out on a Facebook Forum and these are some of the other great responses that I got!

- See all the Major League Baseball parks. Currently there are 30 parks that are being played on with 2 formerly used ones standing (the Astrodome in Houston, and Olympic Stadium in Montreal, Canada (now used as a soccer stadium) (Major League Baseball Parks, 2016).
- See all the National Football League stadiums. Currently there are 32 teams that use 31 stadiums that are being played on (Jets & Giants share). The newest NFL stadium is U.S. Bank Stadium in Minneapolis, Minnesota, home of the Minnesota Vikings, which opens for the 2016 season. You would think that Lambeau Field in Green Bay would be the oldest stadium (built in 1957), but actually Soldier Field in Chicago has been around since 1924 (National Football League Stadiums, 2016).
- National Parks: currently there are 59 National Parks. Yellowstone was the first park to receive NPS status in 1872. I found it interesting that when Yellowstone was established Wyoming, Montana, and Idaho were territories, not states. For this reason, the federal government had to assume responsibility for the land, hence the creation of the national park system (National Park Service, 2016). In the middle of 1986, the National Park Passport Stamp book was published. Travelers take this book to every national park that they go to and get a Park, City, and Date stamp (National Park Passport Stamp, 2016).
- Two other big hits are wineries and microbreweries! According to Wines and Vines, there are more than 9436 wineries in North America, which is up almost 20% from the 8,000 in 2013. While

most of them are in California, Washington, Oregon, New York, and Virginia round out the top 5 states (Klingensmith & Gordon, 2016). In the beer count in July 2013 there were 1165 Brewpubs, 1221 Microbreweries, and 97 local craft beers. In July 2016 there were a total of 1650 Brewpubs, 2397 Microbreweries, and 178 local craft beers. That is a 42% increase in Brewpubs with a 97% & 84% increase in microbreweries and local craft beers (Craft Brewing Statistics, 2016).

- Lighthouses: There are hundreds of lighthouses all around the United States with Michigan having the most at 150. Most of these were built by the United States Coast Guard, and are now protected by the National Lighthouse Preservation Act of 2000 (Lighthouses In the U.S., 2016).
- Covered Bridges: According to sources there are about 1600 covered bridges in the world. Some of the most famous ones can be found right in the Heartland of America: the bridges of Madison County, Iowa. These were made famous by the book and movie of the same name, *Bridges of Madison County*. Bridges for world travelers can be found in China, Canada, Switzerland, Germany, and the United States (Covered Bridges, 2016).
- Other interesting goals I found was to be able to ride a motorcycle year around, play golf year round, hike the mountains, bike the mountains, ski the mountains, working in all the major trauma centers in the United States, and collect the flat "memory" coins from each state.
- Professionally, I have had many nurses and therapists that are in search of "the perfect" place to live. Having a great job in a great community seems to elude most of us. As another nurse states, "To find a hospital and staff that are actually supportive, good teamwork, provides care that makes sense and where I can be proud to work. Physicians, respiratory therapists, and other nurses work collaboratively. I have been doing this for 15 years and haven't found it yet." I personally have been traveling for 13 years, and I have yet to find a hospital that I love in a community that I couldn't live without.

Conclusion

It takes a special type of person to be a nurse, and now travel nursing brings a whole new different aspect to nursing. On top of that, travel nursing is a different animal all itself. I'm all for better patient care and easing the nursing shortage, and that is why I take my turn helping out those hospitals in need. I don't get bored in the same old routine because I change hospitals, and even floors, every three to six months. No, travel nursing is not for everyone, but after reading this book you can make a more informed decision on whether or not travel nursing is right for you.

*** References ***

Travel Nursing Jobs. (2016, July 16). American Mobile, Aureus Medical Group, Cross Country TravCorp, Freedom Healthcare Staffing, Freedom Healthcare, RN Network, and TaleMed.

Institute, K. H. (2011). *KPMG's 2011 U.S. Hospital Nursing Labor Costs Study.* USA: KPMG.

Covered Bridges. (2016). Retrieved from Wikipedia: http://en.wikipedia.org/wiki/Covered_bridge

Craft Brewing Statistics. (2016, July). Retrieved from The Brewer Association: http://www.brewersassociation.org/pages/business-tools/craft-brewing-statistics/number-of-breweries

Klingensmith, C., & Gordon, J. (2016, 01-22). *North American Winery Total Passes 9436*. Retrieved from Wines and Vines: http://www.winesandvines.com/template.cfm?section=news&content=163718

Lighthouses In the U.S. (2016). Retrieved from Wikipedia: http://en.wikipedia.org/wiki/List_of_lighthouses_in_the_United_States

Major League Baseball Parks. (2016). Retrieved from Wikipedia: http://en.wikipedia.org/wiki/List_of_Major_League_Baseball_stadiums

National Football League Stadiums. (2016). Retrieved from Wikipedia: http://en.wikipedia.org/wiki/National_Football_League_Stadiums

National Park Passport Stamp. (2016). Retrieved from Wikipedia: http://en.wikipedia.org/wiki/National_Park_Passport_Stamps

National Park Service. (2016). Retrieved from Wikipedia: http://en.wikipedia.org/wiki/National_parks

Chapter Two

Traits of a Quality Travel Nurse

"Choose a job you love, and you will never have to work a day in your life." (Confucius)

Any nurse can be a traveling nurse, right? Just like anyone can be a nurse, any nurse can be a traveling nurse. In my 13 years of travel nursing, I have found one definite about travel nursing—either you love it or you hate it. I have not found very many people who are stuck in between.

Travel nurses aren't just nurses who cruise around the United States. They have special qualities about them that make them the best in their field. For some nurses these traits come automatically, and some have to work at them. One thing is for sure, if you are a great traveling nurse, you have to obtain these quality traits!

I posted this question to The Gypsy Nurse Caravan group on Facebook and here are the top nine traits: flexibility, confidence, professionalism, integrity, adaptability, dependability, independence, wanderlust, and adventure. Other traits that were mentioned include: sense of humor, courage, relatability, personality, curiosity, fortitude, self-respect, diligence, honor, patience, tolerance, resourcefulness, maturity, and humility.

Flexibility

"The capability of being bent without breaking," is how Webster's defines flexibility. The truth of the matter is, if you can't be flexible in floating, shifts, scheduling, and housing, don't even think about travel nursing. It's the point of breakability that is so individualized!

In many hospitals, the traveler is the first to float. The floor that you are floated to is the point that can break you. To protect yourself, always ask in the interview how much floating you will do? And to what floors? When I was in Tennessee, I floated from telemetry to ICU overflow and ER only about 10% of the time; when I was in Florida, I floated from telemetry to the ER 50% of the time; as a supervisor here in California, I float the ICU travelers to telemetry floor about 90% of the time.

I don't mind floating 10% of the time. I'm the travel nurse. I'm supposed to be willing to float. I really didn't even mind floating to the ER 50% of the time from Telemetry floor when I was in Florida. The people I worked with on both floors were great and I enjoyed the change. In fact, my husband and I made a game of it "betting" on if I was going to work that night on the telemetry floor or in the emergency room.

The last few hospitals that I have worked at as a nursing supervisor, the ICU staff are floated from the ICU to Telemetry about 90% of the time. Unfortunately, some hospital systems have a routine of hiring ICU travel nurses and then floating them to Medical/Surgical or Telemetry floor.

Floating 90% of the time would be my breaking point. I asked some of the ICU nurses if they knew that they would be floated. Most of them stated that they knew about the possibility of floating, but didn't know that they would be on Telemetry floor almost every day. This would be a problem for me. As an ICU nurse, I wouldn't want to lose my ICU skills by working telemetry floor. Not that working telemetry floor is "bad," but you don't have all the higher level of critical thinking for all the drips, ventilator settings, and arterial line experience.

It is also important in floating that you only float to units of competency. My previous experience (before traveling) was in medical, surgical, rehab, psych, and then emergency room. My first travel assignment was in the ER, and I found that I didn't like traveling as an ER nurse. At my little hospital in California, we had standing orders and therefore, autonomy. We could use our professional judgment and start the chest pain protocol while the physician was on his way from a sleep room in the hospital. When I went to "the big city" of Phoenix, we had to ask the doctor for everything. I couldn't even do an EKG on a chest pain patient until the physician saw the patient. So, I took a telemetry job and absolutely loved it. So floating from telemetry to lower level ICU and ER was not a big deal for me, but being floated to the dialysis floor or oncology floor was my breaking point.

It is important that you discuss with the house supervisors the floors that you absolutely cannot be floated to. Always start the conversation with, "I don't mind being floated to MICU, SICU, or CCU, but I am not comfortable working telemetry or med/surg." It is important to put into your contract your areas of competency. I have yet to have a travel company refuse to put into my contract the floors I can and cannot float to.

You must start this process in the interview with the hospital. Not only is it important to discuss the percentage of time that you will be floated, but also what floors you will float to. Then in your contract you put in a paragraph that reads, "As discussed with the manager, I am willing to float to other floors of competency. I will not be required to float to dialysis, renal, OB, or OR." If the list is shorter, you can put down the floors that you are competent to float to. "As discussed with the manager, I am willing to float to medical, psychiatric, telemetry, rehab, ER, step-down, and PACU."

What shift do you usually work? I have worked night shift primarily for the last 20 years. Will I work day shift? Yes, but I want to know ahead of time that is the shift I'm agreeing to. One of the things that I'm seeing more and more in job listings is the day/night rotation. This is my breaking point. Maybe working 8 hours and floating between evenings and nights or even floating between days and evenings wouldn't be bad, but working 12 hours and floating between days/nights is really hard.

Make sure that you put in your contract that you are contracted for the exact time that you will be working. If you can do the day/night rotation, more power to you, but I would definitely ask for a few more dollars an hour to do this! Remember, anything is negotiable!

What is your schedule going to be like and does it matter to you? I don't mind working every weekend or 2 days here and there, but don't schedule me for every other day. That just drives me nuts! I have found a trend in that the younger travelers want all their days in a row. In fact, I've heard of some travelers doing 7 days on and 7 days off. When I was in Phoenix, I still had my home in Lake Havasu City, and I loved my 3 on, 1 off, 3 on, then I spent 7 at home. But when I'm not close to home, I would just have my 3 days in a row, or at least 2 days in the middle of the week and 2 days on the weekend. Some of the older nurses I have found also like 2 days then a random day then 2 days and another random day. What every nurse needs to think of is what you can be flexible with, and what you cannot safely handle and put this in your contract!

Housing is another area that you might have to be flexible with. The best housing that I ever had was a 3 bedroom 2 bath house on a hill on the Oregon coast that was a vacation rental. My family and I have stayed in everything from the vacation rental in Oregon, to a motel room on the lake in North Dakota, to corporate housing in Phoenix.

Things that effect your housing options may be the fact that you travel with pets or family. When my husband and son traveled with me, we had a two-bedroom apartment with utilities, including cable for television and Internet until we decided to get a recreational vehicle (RV).

If you are single, do you want private housing or do you want to save money and live with a roommate? Does the hospital have its own housing? One hospital system that I know of owns its own apartment complex to house the travelers. Another hospital that I have traveled to housed the travelers on a floor that wasn't currently being used. Do you prefer the company handling the housing or do you want to do things by yourself with the housing stipend? The housing coordinator, which may be your recruiter, needs to know exactly what type of housing you are looking for.

In the beginning of travel nurse time, 1980's, the trend was for companies to put travelers into shared housing. You would have a 2 bedroom house or a 2 bed motel room that you stayed in. Travelers really didn't like that idea; therefore, in the 1990's and 2000's, the big thing that every travel company advertised was private housing! About 2010, we started to see this shift to people taking the stipends and finding their own housing related to the fact that the housing companies were providing was substandard. There was also a belief that some companies had allotted a certain amount of money, say $2000/month for housing, but only spending $1500 and pocketing the rest instead of giving it back to the traveler in per diems or salary.

As time moved on, apartment complexes either didn't offer 3-month leases or charge outrageously high prices for a 3-month lease. There was also a trend of hospitals and nurses cancelling contracts for all sorts of reasons, leaving thousands of dollars stuck in a lease. At the same time, pet deposits and pet rent sky rocketed, and apartment became too big of a risk for some nurses. That is when we started to see the RV trend greatly increase. Travelers started catching on to the idea that the stipend will pay for an RV payment and lot rent with some left over, leaving the traveler with money to pocket.

Unfortunately, travel nurses are not immune to housing disasters. Yes, you need to be flexible with your options, but gunshots and cockroaches are on my "No Go" list! I'm okay with non-luxury housing but filth is my breaking point! If you get to your assignment only to find that housing and things are bad, you have every right to call your recruiter and tell them about it! Be flexible, but don't put yourself in danger. Send a picture of a roach to your recruiter at 5:00 p.m., and you're guaranteed an immediate callback or you need a new recruiter!

Commuting long distances is another deal breaker. I don't mind housing that is 20 to 30 minutes away, but I'm not driving an hour or two from my housing to the assignment location. This is especially important if you take an assignment in a larger city. After you arrive and get settled into the apartment, always make a maiden voyage to the hospital. How long does it take? Are you traveling on a freeway that is congested in the morning traffic? Talk to your recruiter as soon as possible to resolve any issues.

If your company doesn't have one, I would find a copy of a move-in/move-out inventory. Be very specific on what you find wrong with the apartment. Is there a ding in the bedroom door? Make sure that it's on there! Even put the little things, like a black mark on the wall. Most important… take pictures!

Confidence

The basics of confidence include knowing your abilities (strong or weak), being confident in your abilities, and being able to take criticism of your abilities. In the travel nursing world, it really is a jungle out there, and that jungle isn't always rainbows and waterfalls. There are big cats that stalk you, snakes that will want to squeeze the life out of you, and gorillas that want to stomp you in the ground.

The skills checklist is a great way to take inventory of your nursing skills. You want to look good to a hospital, but you don't want to "pump up" your skills checklist. This is the time to be truthful with yourself on what you really can and cannot do. If you have never worked with an intracranial pressure monitor don't put that you have lots of experience related to the fact that you have read every article on ICP monitoring but no actual clinical experience. By misrepresenting yourself, you are not only putting your license in danger, but you are also putting a patient's safety in danger.

There is a fine line between being a "know-it-all" and having confidence in yourself. You must prove yourself with your actions and not your words. Don't tell them all about your experience with arterial lines and balloon pumps, but get in there and show them that you can set one up and monitor it the correct way. The problem all starts when a travel nurse goes into the hospital and announces that they have so many credentials, certificates, and experience that she should just be called, "Super Nurse."

I worked with a nurse who thought that she was better than everyone else because she loved her high level patients with an arterial line, balloon pump and who were always intubated and unconscious. She was too high tech of an RN who was WAY smarter than any of the rest of us. After making the rest of the staff look stupid for a couple of weeks, she was eventually told that the hospital no longer needed her.

Accepting criticism is one of the hardest aspects of travel nursing. Here you are a thousand miles from home and "no one likes you." You have to get past this and make your patients a number one priority.

My two worst assignments both involved being criticized almost to the point of breaking. It really amazes me how you can do the exact the same thing at different hospitals and you're a genius at one and an idiot at the other one. Tough times, yeah, but I probably learned the most from those two assignments.

My first toughie was in Oklahoma. When I interviewed for the job, I was asked if I took care of post cardiac catheterization patients. Sure I have, not a problem. My first cardiac cath patient came back with this piece of green plastic sticking out of their leg... Oh! That is what a sheath looks like. I'd heard of them, but all our patients came back with an angioseal at the other hospital.

From then on, I was known as the travel nurse making all the big bucks but getting all the easy patients because I didn't have any experience with a sheath. I poured myself into my patients and their care instead of listening to all their bickering.

My second worst assignment was in North Dakota, which is really a shame, because I really liked most of the people that I worked with.

During my first two months it was amazing how everyone knew the protocol, but none of them did it the exact same way. Every shift I was told about every little thing that I did wrong; although, I was doing it how the others had oriented me to. Then the nursing supervisor started following me around to catch everything that I did wrong. I started making every effort to stay away from her until one day she attempted to throw me under the bus, and I went to the nursing supervisor about working in a hostile environment.

All this is to say that when you are a traveling nurse, you are taking a chance of being attacked by the hospital staff. That is why it is very important for you to have great nursing skills, be confident, and know when to stick up for yourself. Don't let anyone beat you down to your breaking point.

Professionalism & Integrity

You may think that integrity and professionalism are automatic since we are all have a professional nursing license, but I'm still shocked at some of the things that I see out there in the travel nursing world.

The first step to professionalism is the way you look. It's not mandatory, but having your hair up off your shoulders is a good start. Have it neatly trimmed or pulled back nicely. Make sure that your uniform is nice and clean without wrinkles. I know that should be a given, but you would be surprised at how many times I have seen unkempt uniforms. Remember on your first day you only get one chance to make a great first impression.

Another aspect of professionalism is to not get involved in the unit's politics. After all, isn't that one of the reasons we travel? The easiest way of doing this is by not hanging out at the nurses' station, talking about tummy tucks, boob jobs, and boyfriends. You need to be down the hallway with your patients. Patient care has to be number one.

As a supervisor one of the things that really bothers me is the use of pet names. The patients are not your honey, sweetie, papa, or momma. They have a name, which is usually written on the board at the bedside now. It doesn't take very long to see that the patient prefers to go by Suzie instead of momma.

A readiness to help is another aspect of professionalism as a traveling nurse. I don't want to ever hear a professional travel nurse state, "That's not my patient," or, "They didn't help me." It may not be your patient, but that patient has needs that need to be taken care of, and if you are not busy and can help out, why not? Yeah, we all have those patients who are on the call light constantly. Why not tell the nurse, you'll get it this time? Give the other nurse a break. I have found that usually what comes around goes around.

And what about that professional attitude? Yes, we all have bad days, but we don't have them all the time. Every day, you need to come to work with a smile on your face and an attitude that today is going to be a great day! Yeah, I know, this can change within the first 10 minutes of the shift, but at least you got there with a great attitude. Some mornings and evenings half the battle is getting to work with a great attitude!

The best definition of integrity is, "Doing what you know is right, even when no one is looking." If a pill hit the floor and no one is looking do you pick it up and put it back in the container or do you go get another one? What if it's a narcotic? Is it really worth the effort to find someone to waste it with you and get another one? I know, this seems to be a no brainer, but you would be surprised!

You also need to have integrity when it comes to working with the hospital and travel agency. If you say that you are going to be at orientation on the 11th at 7:00 a.m., you had better be there at 7:00 a.m. ready to fill out more paperwork! If you tell your company that you will have your titers done by the start date, then you'd better get them done and resulted by then. I also expect the same integrity from the hospital and agency. If a travel company tells you that you will get a bonus for completing 90% of your hours, I expect to see that bonus. I don't expect the company to come up with some lame excuse that you just missed it without a full detail of why you missed it. Empty verbiage does not translate into integrity.

If the hospital states that you will float 25% of the time, I expect them to honor that, unless there is a further agreement between you and the hospital that you will float more than that. I expect the hospital to have the integrity to give you the guaranteed hours that you are required to have.

Again, do what is right, even when no one else is looking.

Adaptability

As a traveling nurse, you must be able to adjust oneself readily to different conditions. This is where the ole saying, "When in Rome, do as the Romans," comes into play. So many times, I've heard travel nurses state, "Oh, I don't do it like that, because this is how I learned in nursing school and have always done it that way."

Things change…times change…the process is always getting improved. The newest terminology we hear now is evidence-based practice. In 1992 when I got out of nursing school, we didn't do something related to evidence-based practice, we did it because that is how that particular school had been doing it since the new disposable syringes came out! Now there has been such a great leap into evidenced-based practice and nursing research that's how 21st century nurses have to roll.

Another aspect of travel nursing and adaptability is accepting the cultural differences of the areas in which you travel to. This can be anything from a poor town to a rich city, small town to big city, and different ethnic groups. Social classes are seen in all areas, not just poor towns and rich cities. Some patients expect everything to be given to them the minute they ask for it, and others are very patient and understand that you are very busy, and thank you for taking time out especially for them. The differences in a small town or big city are most often the nurses' choice, and this adaptability is up to you, the travel nurse.

Currently my home base is in a town with a whopping population of 1968 people. In just about all the places I have traveled to, I have been in towns anywhere from 10,000 to under 100K. That isn't to say that I haven't taken assignment in a larger market. In fact, the last 2 winters I have spent in the greater Los Angeles area known as the Inland Empire (Riverside County). There are definitely differences in the population of Southeast Idaho and the population of Southern California!

People in Southern California have a hard time understanding that in my little corner of Idaho, we have 1 African-American family and 3 Asian families, and a Hispanic population of 150. The first winter, we were located in Hemet, CA. In that smaller town, there were a total of 41,324 people with 2,600 African-Americans, 13,785 Hispanic, and 1,707 Asians (City Comparison, 2016). It was just such a reverse shock to them, that some parts of the United States weren't as culturally diverse as other areas. They also couldn't believe that we only have about 8600 (all 3 towns) in our county with almost 2,000 people in my town. In the RV Park that I'm in there are more people than there are in my hometown. Nothing wrong with either lifestyle, but it does take some getting used to.

You also have to adapt to the specialty idea if you are from a small town. At home I worked Critical Access (where I was doing ER, ICU, House Supervisor, Med-Surg, Post-Partum, Rehab, and PACU). It is very difficult to explain to recruiters and interviewing managers exactly what my "specialty" is. Anyone who has worked Critical Access (25 beds or less in a rural area), knows that most of the time, you have to know a little of everything and you can't specialize in anything but quality nursing care! I'm very thankful for my small town experiences; not many house supervisors out there have not only BLS, ACLS, and PALS, but NRP, AWHONN, and TNCC. Coming to a hospital of 100 beds, I had to adjust to doing less bedside care and more supervising and staffing.

No matter what your specialty is, each hospital is different and you must adapt to the new policy and procedures. As stated before, it is so important to do as the Romans when in Rome!

Dependability

Dependability is another great attribute that a traveling professional must possess. This means that you must be reliable and show up when you are supposed to. Part of being a travel nurse is showing up every day and doing your job. Once again, you would think that this is a no-brainer, but you would be amazed at the number of hospitals I have been to that are astonished when I show up and do my job.

At one of my assignments, they had gone through several travelers who did nothing in their spare time except shop online, play games on the computer, or sleep. I got there and they were so impressed that I showed up, did my job, and was a true leader, in that, when I wasn't busy in the emergency room, I helped out the others on the medical floor. No, I'm not a super hero, I'm just someone who actually shows up and works.

Dependability is also shown by showing up to work on time. When you first get to your assignment (if not before in the interview) make sure that you know what time orientation starts and what time report starts. Most shifts are 7:00 a.m. to 7:00 p.m., what time is report? Some hospitals do the 0645 to 0715 for report, while others may have report from 0700 to 0730. If report is at 0645 and you show up at 0700, your first impression may not be the best.

Some hospitals are not the best at letting you know about changes. As a travel nurse, you need to check the schedule at least weekly to see if there are any changes. Another thing that makes you really look good is by being available to trade days on occasion. Personally, I don't usually don't have any connections or big doings going on while I'm on assignment; therefore, I'm pretty open to working whenever. No, you don't need to do this all the time, but even being available to trade a few days a month makes you look very adaptable and by actually showing up, very dependable.

Dependability is staying until your shift has ended. If your shift is not over until 0730 and it takes you an hour to get to the dentist, don't schedule your dentist appointment at 0800, which would require you to leave when day shift got there right at 0700. Again, this may seem to be a no-brainer, but I've seen this over and over with both travelers and staff nurses.

Make every attempt to have all your work done by the end of the shift. Yeah, I know, charting as you go at some hospitals is only a dream. As much as you try to keep up with charting, sometimes you just have to stay a little longer to complete everything. I find this especially true if you work the OB floor. Babies have a habit of coming into the world just before shift change! Staying late to get all your charting done isn't the best of situations, but it does happen.

Don't leave things undone! All hospitals are 24-hour facilities and some things you just don't have time to do. Make sure that the oncoming shift knows if you have things that you haven't completed or if you're an ER nurse, make sure that they know exactly what you have and have not done. "Triage, assessment, and EKG have been done, but I don't have an IV line in yet." Don't make it a habit of leaving things undone, by having the attitude, "I've had enough, I'm done, day shift can do that."

Dependability is also shown by not calling off for any reason. The Garth Brooks show is in town and you didn't realize it before the schedule came out, so all of a sudden you are having "eye trouble" (just can't see coming in to work). The best plan is to make every attempt to trade a day with another nurse. If you have already made it a habit of trading days with the other nurses, then they are more apt to trade a day with you when you would like a day off.

Find yourself in a bad assignment? The appropriate thing to do is talk it over with your recruiter. Although we are contracted nurses, most contracts have it in there that you are an "at will" employee that can be cancelled with a two-week notice.

This concept goes both ways. Are you in an assignment that was misrepresented to you? Talk to your recruiter about the appropriate length of time, give your notice and go on with life. The wrong thing to do is to call off every day until the end of the assignment.

Independence

Independence is the freedom from control or influence of another or others. This means that as a traveler you have to have the ability to work without relying on others to help you every step of the way. For most newbie nurses, the toughest part of becoming a travel nurse is waiting a year or two before beginning your travel nurse career. But it is so important that you can stand up on your own two feet without someone being there to help you every step of the way.

Being independent with confidence also means that you won't let the other nursing staff run over you. Again, we find another fine line between being flexible and being run over. Be flexible and adaptable, but don't let them run over you either. Unfortunately, there are some hospitals that you will find yourself with the worst patient every shift and you will feel crapped on. At this point, you have to be independent enough and stand up on your own two feet to say, "Hey, I've had Mr. Code Brown all this week, is there any way that I can switch a patient with someone?" At any time that you find yourself in a hostile environment, it is also wise to follow the chain of command. Tell your recruiter and try to work things out with the charge nurse. If that fails, go to the manager that is your direct report. You have to stand up for yourself!

Adventure & Wanderlust

Oh the wanderlust freedom of travel nursing. The freedom to pick your destination: mountains in the winter for snow skiing, lakes in the summer for water skiing, becoming a snow bird at the age of 35 instead of 65! The freedom to pick your own culture: living the life in the big city with all its hustle and bustle, going to the country and seeing the stars at night, or living in the burbs with quaint shops and local pubs. The freedom to pick your own work environment: large teaching hospital with opportunities to specialize, smaller community hospital where you have the opportunities to experience other units, or smaller hospitals where you get a wide variety of experiences.

Although you may have limited choices related to your specialty and available assignment by one travel company, you are more than free to check out other travel companies that have an assignment where you want to be. No one can tell you that you HAVE to go to Texas in the summer or North Dakota in the winter. You have choices.

This is what travel nursing is all about! Wandering the country and living the adventure. With travel nursing, you don't have to hike the same old trail. You don't have to play the same old golf course. You don't have to take the same old weekend adventure.

I have a friend who is on assignment now in Phoenix who picks a different trail to hike on her days off. The Blogs and Facebook are loaded with pictures of all kinds of nurses taking all kinds of side trips. This is a top reason that travelers love their lifestyle…the adventure and wanderlust of it all!!!

*** Reference ***

City Comparison. (2016). Retrieved from Home Fair: http://www.homefair.com/real-estate/compare-cities/results.asp?Zip1=83241&Zip2=92545 on 06/21/2016 at 1:45pm.

Chapter Three

How Travel Nurses Need To Behave

"Grant me the serenity to accept the things I cannot change, the courage to change the things I can, and the wisdom to know the difference."
(Serenity Prayer)

Travel nurses are no different than the other nurses in the fact that we should all behave ourselves. The thing that is different with travel nursing is that travelers are stereotyped more than staff nurses. Any behaviors that a travel nurse expresses will be recognized and expected for other travelers. Although this is a short chapter, it is one of the most important in that it affects ALL travel nurses! We need to focus on positive behaviors and just say "no" to the ones that will affect the reputation of a traveler.

When In Rome, Do As The Romans Do

I know that we touched this subject last chapter, but this concept is so important to a traveling healthcare professional! This is the golden rule of travel nursing. Never, ever tell anyone that they are doing all wrong because they don't do things like you do. There are several ways to change a dressing, and, as a traveling nurse, you will learn them all.

As a traveler, one of the most valuable things that you can do when you first get onto the nursing floor is find the policy and procedure manual. Yes, there are basic nursing procedures that never change from hospital to hospital, and with other things there are constantly changing related to the new evidence-based practice guides. One of the policies that comes first to my mind is contact precautions for MRSA and VRE. Some hospitals you need full gown, mask, and gloves. Other hospitals you need only gloves unless you are going to be changing the wound where the MRSA is located or emptying the foley catheter where the VRE is located. To change an IV setting or to hit the restart do you need full gown and gloves? The answer to that can only be found in the nursing policy and procedure.

Again, we are on the fine high wire above the circus. Trying to balance what we know and what the hospital facility's policies are. We don't want to look like an idiot asking every 10 minutes on how to do things, but we don't want to just do something that might be wrong and put our patient into danger. A helpful hint to newbie travel nurses is to buy a copy, or know where there is a copy of the Lippincott Nursing Procedures. As a supervisor, I have found that most hospitals rely on this manual for their nursing procedures; consequently, if you have something that you don't know how to do or need a refresher, it is a great resource. What is even handier is that the 2015 version is available as an eBook for your kindle/iPad so that you don't have to lug around the heavy book.

The one thing that does make it difficult at times is the different way that different nurses at the same hospital do it the "right way," but that's not how others have trained you to do the same routine. You also have to figure out the routine or the procedure ways of the physician, especially if you work in the ER or the OR.

Yes, this is a two edged sword in the fact that you have to do procedures the way that you learned them or have found to work best, but you always be open to change.

Just Say No To Gossip

Okay this has to be one of my biggest weaknesses. There are just some things out in the world of travel nursing that will make you scream and it is so easy to fall into the trap. We all want to interact with our fellow nurses, but we have to be careful not to fall into the trap of gossiping about the other nurses.

People are naturally curious; they want to know what's going on. Don't be a victim to sitting at the nurse's station discussing the new handbag from Louis Vuitton, your new Prada shoes, or what new cosmetic procedure that your best friend had.

The best way to keep your mouth shut is to get back to work. Your number one priority should be patient care and not sitting at the nurse station. The more you do for your patients the less time you will have to sit around and gossip.

This will also give you less time to sit around and discuss salaries for what other traveling nurses are making. The danger with discussing your salary with other nurses is that different companies give different benefits, and while your benefits may be great you might be making less hourly wage whereas another nurse may not have as good of benefits but they will be making more hourly wage. There is just no good way to compare apples and oranges over chips and salsa.

Hit The Floor Running

A big complaint that I have seen on travel nursing forums is the fact that someone didn't get enough orientation. As a traveling nurse, you have to be able to hit the floor running. This is the one of the main reasons why you should have at least one to two years in your field. There is no time to lean on someone else. You have to be able to stand up by yourself.

As a staff nurse, orientation is anywhere from a few weeks to several months at a new place of employment. When you are only planning on being there for 13-weeks, things are greatly accelerated. In Oklahoma City, I had 4 hours of orientation and that was it. The longest orientation that I had as a traveling floor nurse was Florida. It was HCA, therefore, I had a day of hospital orientation, a day of nursing orientation, and then 3 days on the floor. As a traveling house supervisor, the longest was in California. I had one week on days, one week on evenings, one week on nights, then I was in charge of the hospital at night all by myself.

You should expect to be shown where the clean and dirty utilities rooms are, the medication room, the kitchen, and be given any codes to get into those different rooms. Orientation should also entail the general routine of the unit and what is expected of you. In no orientation will you learn everything that you will need to know. In fact, I'm constantly finding out new things during my last week on assignment.

Thinking Fast On Your Feet

As a traveling nurse, you need to have the ability to problem solve while on the run. Critical thinking skills are a must for a traveling nurse.

There are times when you have to figure out the best case scenario. Once again, this is the reason why you need to have more than a year of experience before attempting travel nursing.

Critical thinking skills are a must for travelers related to the fact that you are not going to have someone hold your hand. After a short orientation, you will be taking care of your own set of patients. When there is a change in your patient's condition, you have to be able to recognize the problem and start working towards the solution.

During an assignment you will have to know without being prompted when to use those critical thinking skills. You have to always keep in the back of your mind that you are a visitor and that your actions are going to mean a lot more than words.

I had a situation in Arizona where I took care of a patient that had a CBI (continuous bladder irrigation) going on all night. I found myself spending a lot of time with this patient regulating his irrigation to a "rose" color. After I had completed all my assessments and basic cares, I made the independent decision that my CBI patient was taking up a lot of my time, and to make it easier on both of us, I would do all my charting and sit right outside of this guy's door. To make a long story short, my independent critical thinking to stay near the patient saved my contract. The other traveler who came along after me let the CBI bag run dry and they ended up having to take the guy back into surgery. I worked the next night, and she found herself traveling back home Nebraska after they cancelled her contract.

This is the main reason why hospitals and travel companies won't even look at a nurse until they have had at least one to two years of experience. Being able to think fast takes some preparation and mastering of your nursing skills. You can't think fast until you build up the stamina to do so. You have to devote yourself every shift to making sharper and faster decisions about your patient's care. Always think about what is best for the patient. Rome wasn't built in a day and neither was a great travel professional. You have to be confident and self-sufficient.

Willingness To Go On The Fly

Another trait of a great travel nurse is the willingness to do things at a moment's notice. In fact, this happens frequently in some assignments with the floating aspect. You must be able to walk onto a floor, take your assignment, see what needs to be done and take care of your patient's in a proper manner.

This can also be true at the beginning of an assignment. Not all arrangements for the assignment are made weeks in advance. Unfortunately, hospitals and staffing companies will ultimately find something that needs to be done the week before the assignment. Although a lack of planning on their part doesn't necessarily constitute an emergency on your part, you still need to make every attempt to get things completed as soon as possible. We have to remember that travel companies, hospitals, and nurses are not always perfect.

Masters of Change

Traveling nurses and therapists thrive on change! If you are even just a little afraid of change, then don't even think about becoming a travel healthcare professional.

Every travel nurse needs a plaque on the wall of the serenity prayer. "Grant me the serenity to accept the things I cannot change, the courage to change the things I can, and the wisdom to know the difference."

Some of the things that we can do to cope with change and our continuously changing life style are the following:

- Take time to relax. Too many times we get stressed out between all the titers, test, and paperwork that we forget to relax. It is important to find a relaxation technique whether it's meditation, reading, listening to music, or just veggin' out in front of the television.
- Get out and be active. I love it when I see people online getting together to do fun things like hiking, biking, and golfing while on assignment. It doesn't have to be a sport either! Try going out to eat or seeing a movie with another traveler on assignment in your location.
- Remember to take care of yourself. This is one tough thing for nurses. We take care of others really well, but seem to fall short when it comes to taking care of us. Make every attempt to get out and walk for 30 minutes and try to eat healthier. Cheeseburgers and pizza aren't bad, when taken in moderation!
- Kill them with kindness at work. I cannot say it enough; you only have one chance to make a first impression. Go in with a

great attitude and show them that you are there not to change them, but to work and help out.

- Guard yourself with a support system. There are several great groups on Facebook that allow travelers to vent their feelings. If you don't feel comfortable in a group, find a smaller group or a person or two that you can chat with when times get tough.

Powering Through When Times Get Tough

Even at the best of assignments, I've had a tough day to get through. No one said that travel nursing was a field of roses all the time. It can be very demanding and trying at times. You will find yourself in situations when you power through the day or maybe you have to power through the entire 13 weeks.

You have to have the ability to bounce back from adversity. Not everyone is going to be your friend at a new location. When things get tough, the tough get going! You have to meet the adversity head on and tackle the tough jobs. If it's a problem with a co-worker, remember to kill them with kindness and keep on smiling.

Focus on the tasks at hand. You are there to help out in the time of crisis. If things were perfect at that hospital, they wouldn't need travel nurses. Your task is to go to a location and make a concentrated effort to help out in any way you can, on the days or nights that you are scheduled. The reward of doing a great job at work is all the adventures that you will have on your days off. Some days you just want to give up, but you have to keep on focusing until the end of the shift, the end of med pass, the end of the hour.

Keep your eye on the end target. When you get into a bad assignment or even just a bad day, just keep on thinking about the end. Only 10 more weeks, only 5 more hours… In most cases, we can do anything for 13 weeks. One of my toughest assignments was a 20 weeker in North Dakota, in which some days I definitely counted down the hours until the end of the shift. I made it through those 20 weeks, but it was a toughie! That is why it's so important to have a great recruiter that can help you power through the tough times.

Don't forget to trust in yourself. You are a great nurse and you know it! You didn't spend all that time in nursing school and pass state boards just to be a dummy. You have worked hard to get to the point of being a travel nurse. Believe in yourself and don't lose that confidence.

Personalities In Travel Nursing

The personality of a great travel nurse should include one that is outgoing and spirited. If you are shy and meek, you will be run over like a matador during the running of the bulls at the festival of Sanfermines.

That's not to say that you have to be bouncing off the walls, but you do have to be able to stand up by yourself and take up after yourself. You have to have a strong personality that can stand up in the face of diversity.

This is another subject that is a favorite of mine, the personality between the travel nurse and the recruiter. If you and your recruiter have very different personalities, you may need just to switch recruiters instead of changing companies all together.

I think that so many times the biggest problem we have in nursing field is the different types of personalities that we work with from patients, to families, to co-workers and even managers. Again, being a travel nurse is an advantage to the personality game in that if we can't stand the personality of a co-worker or recruiter, we do the best we can for 13 weeks and then we change hospitals and/or recruiters!

In Conclusion

Travel nursing is a very rewarding career, but you definitely have to be the "travel nursing" type or you are going to be miserable. Not a bad nurse, just not happy with the lifestyle. It is very important for nurses to understand what it takes to be a travel nurse before thinking about hitting the road.

Chapter Four

The Good, the Bad, and the Ugly

"Along the fairways of life, you must stop and smell the roses; for you only get to play one round." (Ben Hogan)

This is one of my favorite quotes from the great golfer, Ben Hogan. What does this have to do with travel nursing? The road traveled has many rewards, but it also has its thorny drawbacks and it can throw us completely off-course with an ugly disaster.

Some of the good things about travel nursing include: making new friends, getting a feel of a city before making a move, enhancing your resume, better pay for travel nursing, and getting to eat all the great regional food. The bad include housing nightmares, politics, leaving friends and family behind, obtaining all those state licenses, and starting at a new hospital with little orientation. Then it gets ugly with moving every three months, being lonely, staff grudges, sick days which cost you big time, and getting a contract cancelled.

Making New Friends

When you walk onto the floor everyone is sizing up the new traveler. They want to know how long you have been a nurse, how long you have been traveling, and of course, where you are from. This scenario also works in reverse. One of my first objectives is to find out who is traveler friendly. After 13 years of traveling, the one thing that brings me the most anxiety is the fear of the unknown co-worker. Every time I'm introduced to someone new, I find my mind asking, "Is this going to be the one that I'm going to connect with?" I have yet to have an assignment, even in the worst of assignments, that I haven't made a special connection with someone as a great resource. This is someone who is traveler friendly and seems to be genuinely concerned about making your travel nursing assignment a good one.

Now that we have Facebook, with every assignment my friends list gets bigger and bigger! Except for a few assignments at the beginning of my career, when Facebook wasn't around, I have at least one or two of the nurses from each assignment that I'm still connected with.

With the event of social forums our network of other traveling nurses is also growing. In fact, through one of the longest running groups, Traveling Nurses & Therapists on Delphi Forums, I have met some of the best travelers that have turned out to make a big difference in the world of travel healthcare.

It was from this group that some traveling nurses and a respiratory therapist/tax guru got together with an idea to create a conference on travel nursing. From that group, Michelle, Candy, Phil, Joe, and I are now the directors of the biggest gathering of traveling nurses once a year at the Travelers Conference. With the latest edition of committee members, Cynthia Kinnas, retired recruiter/company president, and Laura Latimer, traveling therapist, this group has come full circle!

Making a big move?

Some nurses use travel nursing as a way to explore where they would like to permanently relocate. If you have hesitations about moving to Phoenix, Minneapolis, Seattle, Boston, Los Angeles, or New Orleans, getting a travel assignment there is a perfect opportunity to test out the waters.

By doing this, you learn a lot about what parts of the city are best for you and your family. This can be done in the larger markets by working short 8 to 13 week assignments at different locations in the city. Not sure you want to stay in Phoenix? Take a break and find a summer assignment in Minneapolis or Boston!

Do you prefer a small town, suburb, or big city? This can also be explored with travel nursing. I have always lived in towns 10,000 people or less. Do I take assignments in the city? Yes, but I usually find myself out in the suburbs. Would I ever work a downtown assignment? Yes! Why? Because I truly have never lived the city life. In fact, one year, I looked at an assignment at the University of Utah in attempt to try out the city life. In exploring the community and surrounding area, we found an apartment close to the facility where I could take the bus to work every evening and then back in the morning. I have one travel nursing friend who has always lived in the city with mass transportation, and doesn't own a car or even have a driver's license. She gets along fine, but not having a car would drive me nuts! Travel nursing gives me the opportunity to try out that lifestyle.

Enhancing Your Resume

One of the biggest misconceptions about travel nursing is that your resume is going to look like you're unstable related to the fact that you have had 14 travel assignments in 5 years. On the contrary, what this points out to someone who is looking for a temporary nurse is that you are very adaptable to different situations.

Along the travel nursing highway you will also have plenty of opportunities to expand that resume. My assignment in Florida is a great example of that. I was working telemetry floor, but had some small ER and small ICU background. When they needed someone to float to ICU, I was the first to go for "step-down" type of patients, patients that would be transferred from ICU to Telemetry the next day, until the day that I walked in and the ICU nurses were bickering about who was going to float to the ER. They had floated me to ICU to have one of the ICU nurses float to ER. It was then that I spoke up and volunteered to go to the ER. I went to the ER and took off just like riding an old bicycle. Telemetry, ICU, or ER? In the end, this was a great assignment related to the fact that the next 13 weeks, I was chosen to open up the admission unit, where all we did was admit patient's from the ER to Telemetry or Medical floor. My resume then expanded to ICU Float and Admission Unit.

I'm frequently asked by travelers if they can "switch" specialties while on assignment. As a traveling nurse, the easiest way to do this is to take a permanent job at a local hospital and get a year's worth of experience in the new specialty. Given a greater amount of time, this can also be done while traveling by floating to increasingly more difficult floors. I'm not suggesting going from telemetry to ICU, but instead an assignment in step-down and offering to help in ICU.

When I was in Tennessee, I frequently floated to ICU to take the low acuity ICU patients. I was considered a "secondary" ICU nurse, which means that I always had a primary ICU nurse as a resource when needed. Most of the time, this was the charge nurse who helped with things that I wasn't familiar with. In Mississippi, I was offered the chance to switch to ICU if I would stay there for a year. The most important factor is not making a big jump, but be aware of smaller jumps that can enhance your resume. Always ask yourself, "Am I putting the patient in danger by taking this float assignment?"

Better Pay

One of the biggest misunderstandings by hospital staff is that travel nurses are making the big bucks. It's true that our bill rate (what the hospital pays) may be higher than what the other nurses are making, but staff nurses don't always understand that we are not pocketing all of the bill rate.

On average, a smaller to medium company will take 10% to 20% of the bill rate for overhead costs, insurance, benefits, etc. I have also found the larger publically traded companies may take 20% to 30%. And, if you are working through a subcontract, your company is usually pocketing 20% while the vendor is pocketing 5% of the bill rate. Not only do staff nurses not understand this fully, but some travel nurses are totally confused about the bill rate.

My personal best example of this goes back to Oklahoma City and a miscommunication. When I interviewed for the job I was asked, "Have you taken care of post cardiac cath patients?" Needless to say, this ended up being a trick question! Yes, I had taken care of post cardiac cath patients, but all of our patient's came back to the floor with a 2x2 and tegaderm over an angioseal. My first post cardiac cath patient in OKC came back with a green piece of plastic sticking out of his leg. My thought: "This is what a cardiac sheath is." That is when I learned that the patients on this floor came back with sheaths, and it was my job to figure out their ACT and when to pull the sheath, which was totally foreign to me. Upon letting the manager know that I didn't pull sheaths, I was automatically labeled as the travel nurse making the big bucks that got the easy patients (didn't have to pull sheaths). Now, by the end of the contract I learned to pull sheaths, but it was 13 weeks of hell (which didn't make sense because I was always willing to be the second RN with my ER background).

Then we get to the discussion of knowing your bill rate and knowing if the travel company is cheating you. There has only been one assignment that I have known my bill rate, and upon doing the calculations, I found that I was losing only 20% on a subcontracted assignment. I was making 80%, my company was making 15%, and the vendor management system was making 5%. This all sounded reasonable to me.

Then you look at what the nurses are making. I know that the C.N.A.s and Unit Secretary's in California are making what I made at home in Idaho as an RN. In one place, the RNs were making between my bill rate and my take home. For example, my bill rate was $60, and I was bringing home $48, and a lot of the nurses were making between $50 and $55 per hour. The only big advantage that I had was all the tax exemptions because I'm a traveling nurse with a tax home. Am I getting a fair deal? Maybe so, maybe no, but the bottom line for me is that my take home for one week is the same as my take home every two weeks back in Idaho. Yes, I have housing coming out of that, but I'm also getting an extra non-monetary bonus in the adventure factor.

My point is…don't look at someone else's bottom line. What do you need to live comfortably? What do you need to have monetary wise to make ends meet? The pay is better, but it's not always monetarily… you have to look at your assets in lifestyle.

Regional Food

This may be the best part of travel nursing…finding where all the good food is! San Francisco is known for their clam chowder and the best chowder, of course, is found in a sourdough bread bowl. There is nothing like a trip down to Pier 49 and having clam chowder in a sourdough bread bowl, but what other kinds of food can you find in the local region?

The Northwest is best known for Seattle's Best Coffee and Starbucks. But what about other local flavors? You are truly missing out if you don't go by Salty's for the best seafood or shopping at Pike's Market for the best local salmon and local clams.

The East is famous for the shrimp burgers that can be found in North Carolina, Brunswick Stew, Boston Baked Beans, and of course you need to have a "dog" when you are on Coney Island.

Florida is best known not only for its key lime pie, but other tropical and swamp favorites such as mango chicken and fried alligator. When in Miami you have to try out the local Cuban restaurants. Fried plantains are the best!

In the south you will find a great combination of fried chicken, mashed potatoes, gravy, and cornbread, along with some fiery Cajun jambalaya, etouffee, and blackened catfish.

The Midwest is known for its homegrown corn and beef. Some of the best barbeque can be found in the Kansas and Missouri regions, along with the best steaks coming out of Nebraska. And if you are in Iowa during the state fair, don't forget to visit the cow made of butter!

A trip to the Southwest will bring you the best in Tex-Mex, chilies, burritos, and other flavors with a kick, which are influenced by our neighbors to the south. In Phoenix, we also found the best in Greek food!

Housing Faux Pas

Life is like a box of chocolates, you just never know what you are going to get. The same with travel nursing housing. In my 13 years, I have done everything from a hotel with a refrigerator and microwave, to an extended stay with a kitchenette, to a studio apartment, to a one bedroom apartment, to a 3 bedroom, 2 bath house on Tillamook Bay.

Sometime there is a big difference in what you NEED in housing and what you WANT in housing. In North Dakota, my husband and I survived the winter in a fishing cabin on the lake with a refrigerator and microwave. I had also brought my small 2 person crock pot and we bought a microwave pasta maker, so we were good for the 5 months we spent there. In our 3 bedroom house on Tillamook Bay we not only had the crock pot and microwave, but a fully furnished kitchen with an outdoor grill. Just goes to show you that housing can be different on every assignment!

This is where communication with your travel company plays an ultimate part in your happiness as a traveling nurse. Did I know about my glorified motel room in North Dakota at the fishing resort? Yes! Did I plan for it…yes! Did I know about my house on the bay on the Oregon Coast? Yes! Did I plan for it…yes!

Housing can take many shapes and sizes. It is your responsibility as a traveling nurse to find out exactly what the company is providing and what is available in that area. With my husband traveling with me, we need something more private, but with single nurses traveling alone, sometimes a sublet or roommate situation is best.

A big trend lately is to take the stipend and get your own housing from www.craigslist.com, www.airbnb.com and www.VRBO.com (vacation rental by owner), or www.corporatevacationbyowner.com. When using these sites, be very careful about people who want you to wire the money, or just seem "fishy." Craigslist is getting really bad about having scammers on there. In fact, if you are going to find your own housing, it is best to get a motel room for a week until you find housing for the 3 months.

Taking the housing that the company offers is also an option. While traveling, I always took the housing that the company offered. This isn't to say that I didn't assist the housing department in finding my own housing (that is how I got the 3 bedroom, 2 bath on the bay in Oregon.)

Now I have realized that the best housing option is a travel trailer! I truly believe that if you are thinking about long-term travel nursing, you really need to think about a home on wheels. Whether it is a small travel trailer for one, a larger one for two, a fifth wheel for the family, or a motor home for the single traveler, RVing is really the way to go for long term traveling. No matter where you are, your home is always in your rear view mirror!

Politics

Politics is the number one reason why nurses turn to travel nursing. In fact, that is the exact reason why I started travel nursing then went back to it 10 years later after a 2-year break. In 2003, I was passed over as a house supervisor related to the fact that they had no one to take my place on the rehab floor. Again in 2013, I was passed up as a director of nursing related to the fact that they had no one to take my place on night shift. Both times they had to replace me because I quit and went on the road.

As a traveler, you do not have to worry about who is going to get the unit manager position, who is going to be the next house supervisor, or who is going to get the holidays off. If I want the holidays off, then I just make sure that my contract ends on December 15th and schedule my next assignment to begin on January 15th.

The politics of travel nursing include choosing the right company and choosing the right hospital. Every company that you talk with thinks that they are the best company out there. The truth of the matter is, a company that may be right for me, may not be right for you. I don't know of any one company that someone has not had a bad experience with. Same goes with hospitals. The ER may be wonderful at the hospital, but the Medical floor may be a total terror.

All the testing that goes on is another form of politics along with all the Associations that have come up. We will be talking about these things more in depth (PBDS, BKAT Joint Commission, NATHO).

Going Away

Leaving an assignment can be very difficult also. I'm sure we all have had those assignments that we just clicked in, and have even thought of staying on full time. These are usually the assignments that we end up extending six months or more. For instance, my assignment in Iowa was only 3 months in length related to the fact that they found someone else to take my place as a night nursing supervisor. This assignment was very hard to leave! After all, I had made several friends, and the job was very rewarding. I really enjoyed my time there, but in 3 short months that was all gone. I found every excuse to get them to let me stay there, but I also knew that my time there was done.

And now we have the Facebook Factor! This really has made leaving an assignment easier. My North Dakota assignment was not the best of situations; in fact, it was my second to the worst assignment in my 13-year career. But, the truth is, I made some amazing friends in a not-so-friendly environment.

At times it is very hard to leave, but you have to just keep your chin up and think of all the friendships that are yet to come.

Obtaining States' Licenses

One nuisance is the time that it takes to get a new license in each state, and then having to decide whether or not to renew that license. What used to take a few hours to fill out and send in now sometimes can take days if you have to work with a police station that only does fingerprints on a certain day, and time consuming if the local place to get photos is 60 miles away. Not tough to do—just time consuming. And then, instead of renewing one license every two to four years, you may have several that need to be renewed, or you may need a new license for the next assignment.

This has become somewhat easier with the creation of the compact licensure system, but not even half of the states are "compact." This is a national coalition of states that recognize each other's licenses. The nurse has to be a resident of a compact state and then she can travel to other compact states without having to get a new license. For instance, since my home is in Idaho, my Idaho nursing license is a compact nursing license. When I went to Iowa, Arizona, Tennessee, and Mississippi there was no need to get a new license; I just gave the hospital a copy of my Idaho license.

I also carry a few other states: California, where I worked for four years, and Oklahoma, where my parents live. When it comes to renewal time, I will have three licenses that need to be renewed (CA, OK, and ID). I have also had licenses in Florida, Oregon, and Washington, which I have chosen to let lapse. I'm 3,000 miles away from Florida, so the chances of me renewing that one is remote, but I have really considered renewing my Oregon and Washington license since I live in Idaho.

That is what you need to evaluate. Do you think that you are going to ever work in that state again, and how close is that state to your home? Another major factor is what does it entail to get that license back from inactive to active? I've heard stories that California can be a bear to renew, so I would never let that one go. As of current, it is taking up to 6 months to renew a license in California. Also, it's taking very long to get a California license verified for transfer to another state. So, therefore, you would really have to think about the advantages and disadvantages of renewing a California or any other state license. In some states, like Montana, you have to verify EVERY license that you have ever had.

Little or No Orientation

For travel nurses, a change is as good as a vacation, but change can also be traumatic to some nurses, especially the "newbies." Nurses start travel nursing because of the excitement and adventure, and then they have to face the reality of catching on quickly and hitting the floor running.

The ideal traveler needs to be able to follow someone one day and take off on their own the next. At times, nursing orientation is as short as a few hours, while other orientations last for a week.

For instance, in Oklahoma City on the intermediate care unit, I had four hours of computer class and four hours of on-the-floor orientation, and then I was on my own. In Plantation, Florida for the telemetry floor,

I had five 8-hour days of orientation, then three days on the floor. Now as a traveling house supervisor I usually have one week to follow the other nurse, one week to split the duties, and one week where I'm on my own with a resource nurse.

In some cases I have had the nursing managers ask me what type of orientation I am used to and go with my style of orientation, but others have their own way of doing things, and that is fine also. Part of being a travel nurse is being a fast learner and going with the flow. You MUST be able to hit the floor running! Personally, I want one day to follow and then let me go, but I know that others would like to have the full three days with someone else.

If you do not feel comfortable after your orientation, you need to talk to your manager about what you don't feel comfortable with, and then learn what you can look for next time to make your orientation go smoother and quicker. Just remember the basics of nursing: assessment, planning, implementation, evaluation, and follow-up.

Moving Every 3 Months

This can be a very ugly problem if you cannot pack lightly. My poor husband…I have to pick on him here. He is a pack rat, and this travel thing has been so stressful on him because he can't find all these "basement bargains" at the thrift store and bring them home. Of course I don't have a problem, since all I bring is all the office stuff and books. Now you know why we had to travel with a cargo trailer at one time! Now we just pack it in the RV. If it doesn't have a place to call home, it doesn't go.

Find out in advance what the apartment is going to come with. Sometimes you will have full linen and kitchen utensils if you are in corporate housing, but if you have an apartment, then these things usually aren't available. That is where the thrift store shopping comes in handy.

Most of the time, though, you will have a dresser, side table, and bed in the bedroom, with a couch and chair in the living room, with a dining room table and chairs in either the dining area or the kitchen. Don't forget to take your vacuum, a television, a microwave, and pot-holders.

What you pack and whom you travel with can also make a difference. When our son was traveling with us, we tended to travel a little heavy. We not only had the office stuff, but hubby had his "workshop" in the front of the trailer to do small repairs, along with all the son's books and schoolwork supplies. Not to mention the fact that we probably had way too many kitchen and cooking items.

A lot of the travelers I have recently met either drive pickups with lockable shells or sport utility vehicles. It can be done in a car by choosing what you take carefully. Also, I have traveled in my car with a topper on. Pack up the topper with non-breakable items just in case it takes a tumble and then pack with care with all the more fragile goodies. Take a first assignment within a few hundred miles to get a good idea of what you need if you require a test run.

Space savers include space bags and rolling instead of folding items! You can also limit your travel items with the plastic container system. You can have one container for the bathroom (a smaller one), one for the kitchen, one for the living room, and one for the bedroom. If it doesn't fit, it doesn't go!

Moving companies are usually too expensive to help you move every time. If you have a family with quite a bit of goodies, it is feasible to hire someone from a temporary agency to help unload your own trailer or a rental trailer, if need be.

Loneliness on the Road

It was the best of times, it was the worst of times, and it was the loneliest of times. Traveling gives you a lot of experience with different cultures, climates, and personalities, but even with all your acquaintances that you meet on assignment, there are still times when you miss your family and friends.

It doesn't matter whether you travel alone or with a family, loneliness will find you. One of the biggest things is to keep in touch with those that matter to you the most. I miss my family in Oklahoma, but have very strong ties in that I call my parents two or three times a week, and my brother every Tuesday. My husband calls his brother usually about once a week.

And then there is social media! With the invention of Facebook, MySpace, Skype, Instagram, and Pinterest, we are always meeting up with our friends and family online! Some of my best moments have been chatting on Skype or Facebook with friends back home in Idaho. It's also become easier and easier to get involved with other travel nursing groups and friends who are in the same area that you are. In fact, Phoenix travelers have their own Facebook page to assist travelers in organizing Meet and Greets. There are also area groups for traveling healthcare professionals, such as Southern California, Northern California, and the Pacific Northwest (Washington, Oregon, and Idaho),

If you live in an RV, meeting up with other RVers is also very easy to do. If you go south for the winter, the parks have all kinds of things going on. If nothing else, sit outside and read a book. Look up on occasion and tell the walker passing by, "Hello." You just never know what kind of conversation is going to come up next!

Then you can also do things the old fashion way by taking time to get in involved in other activities such as a church, friends of the library, or the neighborhood Bunco game!

Sick Days with Charge

Another downside related to money is losing out when you are not feeling so great. Not only do you not get paid for the day that you miss, but some companies even charge you for housing costs, their reason being that they are paying for housing for you to work thirty-six hours a week, and when you don't live up to that obligation, they do not get their money from their hospital bill rate; therefore, they are losing out on income, hence you will lose also.

Some of the smaller companies are starting to let nurses have paid time off and/or vacation pay, but this is a very new concept. Most companies that I have dealt with will require you to make those days up, either during that week or the next week. If a whole week is missed, the days may be added to the end of the contract.

This is one thing that you need to make sure that is clear in your contract. Is there a penalty in there? Once you sign it's a done deal. If you miss a day without making it up, remember that you are the one who signed the contract with the terms.

Staff Grudges

Some of the ugliest situations I have seen are staff grudges. Now that you are making all these "big bucks," some regular staff think that you need to be assigned the most difficult patients, because travelers are there just for the money anyway.

There is also this misconception in some places that the hospital's bill rate (what they are paying out) is also what the nurses are getting; therefore, I have had some nurses want to know if I really do make seventy dollars an hour. They do not understand about the company getting their share and the travel company paying out for housing and other expenses.

Traveler "hostile" hospitals are out there, but they are few and far between. Some nurses have expressed the fact that they get the tough bed assignments because the staff believes that since the traveler makes more money, they can have the group of patients with persistent nausea, vomiting, diarrhea, the gastro-intestinal bleeds, and the Alzheimer's patients.

I have only been in two hospitals where the hospital management wasn't hostile, but the nurses were; and then again, the nurse management was also "relieved of duties" half way through the assignment, in both hospitals!

Cancelled Contract

This is one of the biggest fears of a traveling health professional—having a cancelled contract. Unfortunately, this has become a bigger and bigger concern over the last few years. Hospitals hire more travelers than they can afford and end up canceling someone's contract. This is also where you see the biggest difference between a good travel company and a great travel company. This is why it's so important to choose a traveling company and a recruiter that is going to have your back.

The greatest expense to a company that can directly affect you is having a 3-month lease on an apartment. If you are cancelled, then the company still has a lease on an apartment for 3 months. The best of travel companies will make every attempt to find you something else within driving distance, but if you are in a smaller city with only one hospital, this can be very difficult if not impossible to do. A great travel company in this case would forgive the rest of the lease, but some of the companies who are all about the money will make every attempt to have you pay for the cancelled lease.

This also puts the traveling health professional out of a job and out of a monetary resource. This can be a dire emergency if you don't have enough in the bank to survive up to a month without a job. I encourage everyone to have at least one-month of reserve, and it is most definitely better if you can save up to 3 months' worth of reserve.

This is also the biggest downside to getting your own housing. Then you are completely responsible for the lease, unless you have a super company that will help you out with the rest of the lease.

On the other hand, this is the biggest advantage of travelling in an RV. Usually your space rent is on a month-to-month basis with no lease; therefore, you just pull the slides in and take off to the next assignment!

In conclusion

There are many good things, a small amount of bad things, and few ugly things you should know about travel nursing. Your mission, should you choose to accept it, is to make a list of all the good and bad things that you need to consider to further evaluate if this way of life is right for you.

Travel nursing is definitely an adventure. You just have to be tough enough to take a few bumps in the road.

Chapter Five

Travel Company Fundamentals

"A great advantage of a corporation is supposed to be the large pool of talent in which its leaders can find and groom high achievers and successors."
(Margaret Heffernan)

This will be the first major decision that you will have to make after deciding to go on the road full time. There are quite a number of companies out there, and only by understanding the travel company itself, knowing what you want, and doing a lot of research will you be happy in your travel nursing career. There are quite a few that can get you a job, but only a handful that will give you exactly what *you* want.

One of the first things you need to understand is the structure of the agency that you are working for. You may only be in contact on a weekly basis with your recruiter, but people such as the staff supervisor, housing coordinator, payroll specialist, and quality assurance are some of the others that you will come in contact with.

Recruiter Basics

This is perhaps the most significant person in travel nursing. This is the individual in whom you will confide your every want for your livelihood, and who will attempt to give you everything you desire to make your life the fullest that it can be. This is the liaison between you and the hospital. It is their job to help select the appropriate assignment for you. This is the person who takes your profile for a company and submits it to the hospital.

The latest trend in staffing companies is to rename the recruiter as a "career consultant" or "talent manager." Behind the fancy new names, they are still people who are in the business of bringing nurses together with hospitals. Another trend is to have a recruiter assistant who helps with all the paperwork and finding jobs, but then you have a "account manager" that is the connection between you and the hospital. Ultimately, you will come to rely on your recruiter or staff supervisor to locate the right obligation for you and ensure that all your needs are being met. This is also the person whom you contact if things are not the way you expected them to be.

One of the advantages of staying with the same company that I have found is that your staff supervisor and/or nursing recruiter will come to know your personality and nursing style. By getting to know you better, what you are and where you are headed in your travel-nursing career, they can assist you in finding the right path. Remember that your recruiter should be there to assist you at any time. If not himself or herself, then someone should be on-call for the nursing company.

Your recruiter should be an asset to you and your choices, and not a deterrent to your nursing experience. Your recruiter should want you to feel contented in your new setting. They should be concerned about your safety by not putting you into precarious circumstances. Your recruiter should be a help to you by finding out what you like to do and where you want to go. Your recruiter should know your preferences for a small, moderate, large, or teaching hospital.

This last year I was having a terrible time finding a new assignment, and my recruiter that I have been with for quite a while called me and said, "I know that it is not the location that you really want, but it's close, and I think that you will love the area." Other times she would tell me of jobs, but tell me "I really don't think that you'll be interested in this assignment, but it is available and I just wanted you to know about it." And usually she is right on the money on what I like and where I want to go.

Your recruiter should know your strengths and weaknesses. They should know what areas of the hospital you can work in as a primary nurse and what areas you are able to float to.

The Used Car Salesman

Any recruiter, any person, can "sell" you, but do you really want a recruiter or a "used car salesman?" To prove my point, I did some research on what makes a successful car salesman. After visiting just a few websites on the characteristics of a good car salesman, I was astonished at how many recruiters I have met had these same qualities.

A recruiter must be personable. What do I mean by "personable?" They must be pleasant in appearance and personality. No, you probably will never *see* your recruiter, but what about their telephone appearance? Good telephone skills are a must with any recruiter. They must have a pleasant voice, and be someone that you *want* to talk to, not someone that you *have* to talk to.

A recruiter must be knowledgeable. It is not a crime to not know the answer to your question, but your recruiter must know where to find the answer. In some research on travel nursing companies that I have done, several times I was referred to the human resources director, who promptly answered my questions about benefits.

How much does your recruiter know about the nursing field? He might be able to sell you a car, but does he know more about an oil change or a blood transfusion? I am a nurse because I care about people. I want to help others in their time of need and to help them feel better. Sure, I could give someone blood, but what kind of ethics would I have if I just gave the person any old blood without double checking the patient's blood type and double checking the name band before giving that patient the blood? It is a lot easier to replace the oil in your car than to fix a mistake with a blood transfusion.

I'm not saying that the recruiter has to be a nurse, just that they must have extended knowledge of the nursing field. How can a recruiter help you out when/if you get into a bind if they can't understand what is happening at the time? I just don't see how a recruiter can "go to bat" for you if they don't know what they are talking about. These hospitals are hiring travelers because they are short-staffed. Under these conditions, several things can go wrong. I would absolutely refuse to take a position if I didn't feel like I had support from my recruiter.

They must know their product, as well as that of the competition. In order to acquire new nurses, you have to offer the nurse something better than the other companies do. The only way you can do that is if you know what the other companies are offering. Little things, like just a few more dollars an hour or better insurance benefits, can make a big difference. So what if every assignment has a completion bonus if you are making only $20/hour? Attempt to find out what other companies are giving their employees at the same or a nearby location, and then make the deal just a little sweeter, which brings me to my next point of knowing your "customer."

The first thing out of a recruiter's mouth should be, "How can I help you?" So many times, what the recruiter says is translated into, "How can you help us?" These "headhunters" are out there to rope you in no matter what it takes. They *need* you. They don't have a company without the nurse, but so many think that the nurse needs them more. New cars look very nice on the lot, but a lot of good they are doing the salesperson if they stay on the lot.

The recruiter that is going to get my attention is the one that says, "How can I help you fulfill your needs in your nursing career?" Nurses travel for many reasons. The need for a nurse who is fighting bankruptcy is so much different from the nurse who just bought a new car and has a burning desire to see the world.

Above all, a recruiter must have a great personality. I have yet to see a rude, crude, and socially unacceptable nursing recruiter have very many nurses who work for them. Yes, there are some out there, and unfortunately, some of the nurses that I network with have had to work with them, but I have yet to meet a person who will stay with a recruiter who is always on the down and depressed side.

A great personality also means a nursing recruiter who is not only concerned about the benefits of having you work for them, but also what is in your best interest. Like the company that I work for presently—everyone shares the benefits of the nurses; there is no "fighting" for nurses because of that great commission.

A great personality also means that they will be there for you when you need someone to lean on. When the tough times come, you should be able to pick up the phone and discuss the problems you are having with your recruiter. We aren't going to get along with everyone, and not everything is going to be perfect. I want a recruiter whom I can call and tell that I really don't feel comfortable in my current situation because of even such a simple thing as a personality conflict. I want a recruiter who will weather the storm with me, not jump ship and let me feel like I have been stranded in the middle of the ocean fighting to keep the sharks away.

The Housing Coordinator

After you have selected an assignment, you will then work closely with the housing coordinator. Their job is to make some place your home away from home. Most travel companies have contracts with hotels, suites, and apartment complexes in which you get housing paid for by the company. Housing can include or exclude a roommate, selected by you and/or the company. Most companies pay for up to a one-bedroom apartment. A few of the companies even pay for bigger places for your entire family. And yes, the companies encourage your immediate family to travel with you. A happy traveler is a great worker! The company provides all of this for you, although sometimes you might have to ask for it.

If you already have a place to stay, most companies offer a housing stipend in which they give you a certain amount of money that you can use to provide your own housing. These housing stipends are usually tax-deductible, as long as you use the money for business housing. Many nurses take the stipend and either live with relatives or use it to live in a recreational vehicle.

Housing coordinators make every attempt to find the best housing available for the amount of money that they are budgeted for, according to the bill rate and the housing rate for the area. It frustrates them when something doesn't work out right or they just are not able to provide every stipulation the nurse wants, and then all the nurse wants to do is complain about the housing that they did find. Nurses need to realize that it is sometimes very hard to find exactly what the nurse wants at a price that he or she wants.

The Payroll Specialist

A payroll specialist is responsible for ensuring you are paid every pay period. Most companies make this easier by implementing direct deposit. The money is "zapped" from your travel nursing company right into your personal checking or savings account. Although it is your payroll's or the recruiter's job to put the data into the computer for you to be paid, the payroll specialist is the one responsible for making sure that you get your check at the appropriate time that you are scheduled to be paid. Check with your recruiter or staff supervisor to see whom you will turn to if there is a problem with payroll. Some companies prefer you to deal directly with the staff supervisor and some will have you deal directly with the payroll specialist.

Mike, a payroll controller states, "Payroll in the travel nursing industry is extremely complicated. Some have their housing paid, while others receive monthly housing stipends; travel pay is due on different dates; weekly pay includes taxed income, or some elect to receive a portion of their income tax free; reimbursements for nursing licenses, other applicable bonuses from time to time; hospitals observe different holidays and different hours to receive holiday pay; and notes on timesheets written from travelers are sometimes not legible. You also have to consider the nurse's request for paid time off days and vacation pay. It doesn't appear to be that complicated, but multiply that by several hundred travelers weekly and it becomes very complex!

"With this type of complexity, mistakes can occur. It's what your travel company does about the situation and the response time to correct it that makes a difference. We, like everyone else, make mistakes. We create processes and modify processes each time mistakes occur in order to minimize them from reoccurring. We even go as far as to wire it into our traveler's bank accounts immediately, if it's our mistake, at no cost to the traveler. Some of these mistakes can be avoided by getting timesheets in on time. This permits our payroll department to ensure that your pay is correct before meeting the deadlines to be processed by payroll firms and entered into your direct deposit account in time for you to be paid on time."

Benefits Specialist

You might also come into contact with the benefits specialist. These wonderful people assist you with your benefits from 401K plans, insurance, incentive programs, completion bonuses, and reward programs. Don't be afraid to call them if you think you are not getting all the benefits that you are entitled to. They are very good resources for reliable answers. Unless your recruiter is getting the same benefits as you are, they may not know all the benefits that you are entitled to.

Shirley, a director of administrative services for a national travel nursing company, tells me, "Benefits were made to be used to offset skyrocketing healthcare costs when you need treatment. That is why our organization pays for our travelers' benefits in full each month. We research various insurance companies yearly to ensure that our travelers are receiving the maximum insurance coverage while containing the cost.

"In addition, those who elect to join 401(k) programs need to take the time to read how to manipulate the 401(k) website that's assigned to those who join. You are able to track your investments and returns on a weekly basis, if you choose. Some travelers don't take the time to do their homework. The benefit is clearly to the traveler's advantage, but most don't recognize the value.

"As long as our travelers understand that they have the right to ask and have the right to an answer in a timely manner, we're glad to help them in any way possible. Other free benefits including continuing education, online forms, online payroll stubs, vacation pay, earned paid time off days, and the like make being a traveler less complicated and risky. Make sure that you're able to use these things to your advantage! If you're not sure, feel free to ask. That's what we're here for!"

Quality Control Specialist

Some companies even use a quality control specialist, who is like a human resource department that helps you meet compliance criteria for each of your assignments. The quality control manager will help you in all aspects of getting ready for your assignment. I get a call on every assignment from the quality control manager making sure that my needs are being taken care of by my staff supervisor. In my opinion, this is a *must* for every travel nursing company who wants to have a quality nursing staff. If the nurses are not happy, how can the patients be happy?

Quality Assurance

A few years ago, I spent a lovely morning with the quality assurance team for Trinity Healthcare Staffing and found the girls in the office to be quite pleasant. I sincerely hope that after this section of the book, nurses will have a better understanding of the functions of this department, and that they really aren't the "QA Nazis" some nurses have them labeled as. Instead of being defined as "a person who fanatically seeks to control a specific activity or practice," they need to be thought of as a department that is dedicated to assuring that the quality of the nursing staff is well documented.

Their job is one of the toughest in the industry due to the fact that it is their task is to keep up with what the hospitals must have as far as immunizations, urine drug screens, medication testing, background checks, and other tests that are required, especially if the company is Joint Commission certified.

As I walked into the QA office, I faced a large board with the requirements for several vendor management and hospital associations, through which most travel nursing contracts are processed. Next to each vendor management name was a list of the particular requirements for that state or regional area. No two vendor management companies required the exact same things. Some require only one PPD, while others required two. Others required titers for chicken pox, while others required just a statement that you have had the disease.

Before a job can be confirmed, all of the nurse's ducks have to be in a row in this river of paper. It is the quality assurance analyst's job to make sure that the nurse's paperwork is in line for the job that they are going to accept, and if it isn't, then it's their job to make sure that they get it. Therefore, they have to notify the recruiter of things needed to complete the file, and the recruiters have to "bug" the nurses until all the paperwork is in. Although this can be very annoying, nurses have to realize that this is required from the hospital to the nursing staff company.

Doing Your Shopping

There are plenty of travel companies out there. Do your shopping; do not just grab the first one that makes you an offer. Plan to start looking for a company about a month before planning on going into travel nursing if at all possible. This process will include finding out more about benefits, locations, and general operations of the travel company.

When shopping for a travel company, be aware that some are going to want you to fill out their application and send all of your personal records and qualifications before they will submit you to a hospital. At this point, be careful to give them just your basic information and let them know that you are just shopping for a travel company. Don't make the mistake of filling out applications and checklists for fifty different companies just to interview them.

Also, be careful about who you give your phone number to until you have done your homework. Once you give the travel company your phone number, you will receive phone calls every week, asking you about assignments. It doesn't take long to rack up the minutes on your cell phone. Plus it's a real inconvenience if you work night shift. You will have no other choice but to turn off your cell phone when you want to sleep.

After reading this chapter, you will be able to find the one company that is going to make you happy in the long run. You will be able to find the one company that goes where you want to go. But first, we need to begin the process of narrowing down your choices.

One thing that should be on that list is your wage requirements. In your staff job, you needed a certain amount per hour to live on. With travel nursing, the trend now is to know exactly how much you are going to bring home in a week. You need to know exactly what you need, and not necessarily what you want, to live your new lifestyle. What is the going rate for that area? Check out www.salary.com, you should be making about 10–20% more a week than the staff nurses. Remember now, that the company is taking 15–25%.

What kind of housing do you require? If you are single and fancy free? Is motel or extended-stay sufficient? The positives of staying in a motel is that they usually have laundry facilities, a pool, and of course, maid service! There are some very nice extended stays that will even allow you to have your four-legged family with you.

Most companies will provide a one-bedroom furnished apartment. You just bring clothes, linens, and personal items. Watch this option, though, because some companies will tell you that you have a "private" bedroom, when in reality you have a private bedroom with shared common areas with another traveler. This may be fine for a lonely traveler, but most of us like the privacy of our own apartment. This option definitely does not work out if you travel with your family.

Planning to take your family? Most companies will work with you on that. They will provide a two-bedroom apartment for you, although you may be expected to pay utilities or some of the rent. The most convenient way to travel with your family is in an RV.

What are your location requirements? Do you want to stay in your home state or the surrounding states? With the invention of compact states, you could decide just to travel in compact states. Favorite destinations seem to be Hawaii and Alaska on the west coast in the winter or Maine in the summer, with winter in Florida for the east coast. You might even choose to stay in the middle by going to North Dakota in the summer and to Texas in the winter. Love to ski? Then go snow skiing in Colorado in the winter and to the lakes of Tennessee for water skiing in the summer. The possibilities are endless.

What about other benefits that you should expect out of a travel nursing company? The biggest seems to be health insurance, 401K, continuing education requirements, longevity, and completion bonuses. These things all matter in your decision!

Find the one company who has the appropriate nursing retention program. What kinds of benefits are added on the longer that you are with them? Almost all companies have this, whether it is in lieu of money or fits into a reward program.

Don't settle for a company that does not provide a 401K program. Not only should they allow you to put tax-free money in, but they should also be making some kind of vested contribution.

Make sure that the company is reliable. Once you get "out there" in the big world of travel nursing, there are going to be days where the only friend you have is your recruiter or staffing supervisor.

Keep your list handy in your planning stage. As we explore more about your career as a travel nurse, you may want to add more ideas. Don't forget to put on your list the places where you would like to travel. You will need that information because not all travel companies go to all areas of the United States and beyond.

Doing Your Research

Now that you have your list of benefit requirements, use the up-to-date graph, "The Ultimate List Of Travel Companies," on the website www.highwayhypodermics.com to get an idea of which companies offer the benefits that are most important to you. You will also want to read the chapter in this book entitled "Travel Company Profiles."

Do more research on the Internet by visiting discussion boards and travel nursing forums, and ask other nurses what they think of those travel companies. This is where you will find out the inside information on these companies. There are quite a few boards on Facebook including, "Traveling The Country, One Hospital At A Time," "Travelers and Recruiters Unite", "Our Gypsy Nurse Caravan," and of course the Highway Hypodermics Page. We also sponsor a "Travel Nursing Newbies" group, "RV Travelers" group, and a "Homeschooling Rn Travel Nurses" group.

Be aware that lurking recruiters may be on the discussion boards and travel nursing forums. Not that I would not talk to them, but just beware that the person who is telling you, "Everything is great with this company," might just be working for that company; therefore, you will have a biased opinion. The only discussion board that I know of that doesn't have recruiters is "Traveling The Country, One Hospital At A Time."

The "Travel Nursing" group is full of jobs, "Travel Nursing Made Simple" and "Travel Nursing - Answers and Advice" are both recruiter administrated groups.

After narrowing your decision down to about five different companies that you would like to work for, submit a complete application for employment to these five companies.

Upon receiving your application, a recruiter will promptly contact you. Talk to the recruiter and find out what hospitals they have that you are interested in. Find out how many jobs they have available for your specialty. This is especially important if you have a specialty that is on the "hard to find" list, such as psychiatric, rehabilitation, or pediatric emergency care.

Not only should the recruiter interview you, but you should also interview the recruiter! This is easiest done if you get out a notebook to keep track of the questions that you have asked.

Each entry should list the company's name, address, phone number, and the person you talked to. The next entry should be the size of the company. The smaller companies may not have as great a selection of places to travel to, but the customer service is usually impeccable.

Next, you might want to know what kind of structure their recruiters work with. If the recruiters work on a commission basis, you will have a greater chance of a recruiter wanting to sign you up just to make money off of you. If the recruiter is on a shared commission basis you are more likely to find a company that will be based on a teamwork effort, which is always to the advantage of the travel nurse. This also leads to the fact that some companies cater to the hospital, whereas others cater to the nurse.

You will also want to know what the process is in case you decide to change recruiters. When problems arise, you want a recruiter that you feel you can work with. If you feel like the recruiter isn't working hard on your side, or if there are personality clashes, it is much easier to switch recruiters than to switch companies. You don't want to get attached to a company that is not going to work with you on problem solving. Along with this, you also need to find out if there is a recruiter supervisor and who it is. Sometimes this will be the owner in a small company or a regional supervisor in a larger company.

You will want to know from the recruiter if they can place you regionally, nationally, or internationally. Some companies only cover certain regions, or they have different offices for different regions. Some companies only cover certain states and there are some states that are only contracted with certain companies. If you are interested in traveling internationally, you will want to find a company that specializes in international travel. International travel brings into play a very different set of rules because of immunizations, passports, work visas, etc. In fact, this year, we have a FULL chapter dedicated to traveling internationally authored by an international flight nurse!

You will want to know how many assignments are available with the company. This is especially important if location is your number one priority. If this requirement isn't fulfilled, then you are going to find yourself hunting for a different company for each assignment.

You will need to find out what kinds of specialties are offered through the company. The most common specialty companies that I have found are companies who specialize only in providing hospital operating room personnel. A few companies out there specialize only in providing management personnel. If your specialty is Med/Surg, you will have quite a few companies to choose from, but if your specialty is psychiatric or rehabilitation you might have trouble finding a company who provides those types of jobs.

You need to get out your list of priority benefits and ask about those. Your priority benefit list might include the type of insurance they provide, the name of the company their insurance is with, whether it's a PPO, HMO, or just a major medical plan. What are the deductibles and how much does the insurance cost the travel nurse? Yes, there are companies out there who provide free medical insurance for their travel nurses. This is a question that you have to ask yourself: are you willing to pay a small amount for your insurance?

You will want to know when you will be paid and how you will be paid. Most companies will send you a weekly check, but there are some out there that only pay bi-weekly or monthly. If you receive a housing stipend, find out if you will be paid the stipend on a weekly or monthly basis. Are monthly stipends paid at the first of the month or at the end of the month?

You will need to find out if the company writes guaranteed hours into their contracts. How many hours do you want to work? Some companies will give you a guarantee of thirty-six hours, while others will guarantee you forty-eight hours. Are those hours broken into eight-hour shifts, ten-hour shifts, or twelve-hour shifts?

What lengths of assignments does the company offer? In a fast response situation, you might find assignments lasting only four weeks. At other places, you might find companies that offer six to nine month contracts. For those nurses who are traveling with school-age children, maybe a nine-month contract during the school year would be preferred over a short-term contract.

If you take the housing, then you will want to know what type of housing is available. Are there are any additional costs to the traveler? Will you have to share housing with another traveler? If you take the subsidy, you will want to know if they pay just what your expenses are, or if you get to keep any of the extra money if there is any left over after paying your expenses. The housing subsidy should be equal to the cost of renting a one-bedroom apartment.

Another thing that you might want to know in the company interview is if airfare and rental car fees are provided. This is especially true if you plan to travel somewhere outside the continental forty-eight states, such as Hawaii, Alaska, or the Virgin Islands. Airfare is definitely needed for a trip to Hawaii, but some travel nurses opt out of the rental car fees and purchase a vehicle from other travel nurses who are leaving the island.

Submission Requirements

What is required before you can be submitted to a hospital? With most companies, all you need is an application for employment, a skills checklist, and a resume. Other travel companies will want all the ducks in a row before they will even submit you. If you are sure that you want to go with that company and location, then go for it, but be careful about filling out too many forms for too many companies. This can be very time consuming, and in effect, waste time if you are not serious about working for that company.

After the interview, if you feel comfortable in continuing a relationship with those companies, then fill out other required forms. One mistake I made when I started out was to fill out the checklist and an application with about 30 different companies. Not only did it take several days to do all of those applications and checklists, but my phone wouldn't stop ringing until I actually went on assignment and my home phone number was disconnected.

Personally, I never give out the phone number of my current place of employment. Some recruiters don't care how busy you are; they are out to secure you—"their" travel nurse—and you have the problem of too many phone calls at your current place of business. And yes, whatever company you are looking at, they do have recruiters that work in the evening and at night!

Once you have decided on a travel company you will need to pick a place for them to submit your profile. Be very careful to keep track of what company has sent your profile to which hospital. Your chances at that hospital can be ruined if two different travel companies submit your profile.

Chapter Six

Location, Corporation, and Documentation

"If it's not documented, it's not done."
(All Nurse Educators)

Time to get started looking for your first assignment. In order to have a successful first assignment we must find a great location, the right travel nursing company, the right hospital, and have all of our ducks in a row when it comes to our credentials. This part of travel nursing is very stressful, but it can also be a lot of fun trying to figure out where you want to go and work.

Depending on your specialty the location or the travel company can be picked first. If your specialty is a common one (LDRP, ICU, ER, or MST), then you can pick your travel company first and where you would like to go next. If you are in psych, rehab, or a house supervisor, you are going to have to find the company that has the most jobs at the time, and you will have a narrow field of locations to choose from.

Location

If location is the most important thing to you, you will need to find the travel company that goes where you want to go. Almost all companies now have their jobs posted online. The one thing that you need to watch out for is companies that have posted jobs with a start date of more than 3 months ago. Chances are that company doesn't keep their job listings current.

Another way to find a job in a certain area is to call the hospital and talk to human resources. Ask them which companies they use for the travel nursing contracts. Some hospital systems have their own company or use one of the larger companies. Hospital Corporation of America (HCA) has their own travel company, Parallon, and Kaiser

Permanente in California uses AMN Healthcare to fulfill their travel nursing needs. When these companies can't fill the jobs themselves, then they will subcontract out to the smaller companies.

The next step is investigating the hospital and community that you are looking at. Search the Internet for more information. Search area chat rooms and do a search on a messaging program for people in that area. The Chamber of Commerce and City Website are good places to start.

The best place I have found to gain information about a new location is at www.homefair.com. It is there that you can find information on a cost-of-living comparison, city report, school reports, crime statistics, moving calculator, choosing the right school, and rental furniture. The first place that I start is with the city report. This will give you a good idea of what to expect regarding crime rate, city size, climate, age demographics, and the major employers. There is also www.crimemapping.com that has a list of all the crimes that have occurred in a certain area.

Another excellent source for information is on www.apartments.com. This is especially useful if you are assisting a company in obtaining your own housing. You can also compare what your company is setting you up in to other housing available in that area. For reviews you can check out www.apartmentratings.com to see if there is anyone happy with the place. Just remember to read the comments and don't necessarily go by the rating. Another thing to remember is that people who are upset are more likely to post a rating than a person who is happy with the place.

This brings up another critical element in choosing a travel company: look at, and ask about, the type of housing each company provides in the area that you are looking at. A lot can be told about a company by their housing. Are you getting a deluxe company with a deluxe apartment, or are you getting an older shack?

The companies who really care about their nurses know that a nurse will only be happy if they feel comfortable and safe in their surroundings. Get to know your surroundings online before accepting any job assignment!

Find out what amenities are available at the apartment or motel. Do they have a pool or spa? What about a workout or weight room? Do they allow pets, and if so, how much does it cost for a pet deposit? And, in recent years, is there a monthly pet rental fee?

If you travel in an RV, you definitely will want to find out if there are any RV parks close by that accept long-term visitors. I am finding out now that some of the newer parks will only accept you if your vehicle was made in the last ten years.

I work nights and my husband is disabled; therefore, our two main priorities are a hot tub and a place that is quiet during the day.

If you have a child, you might want to find out about what schools are available or what support systems are available for home-schooled children. I also want to know where the local church is and what kind of teen programs they have.

Now that we have a company and an area that we would like to go to, the next critical step is to investigate and interview the hospital.

Ask yourself, "What type of hospital am I looking for?" Do you prefer a large hospital, a teaching hospital, or a smaller community hospital? Or…does size really matter?

Are you looking to go to a specific region in the country? Make a list of what you are looking for in a hospital. Even though I came from a small hospital, I really enjoyed my time at the level one trauma center that I worked at in Phoenix, Arizona.

Yes, I definitely was more stressed out, but I was treated as a name and not a number. I had a large support system there, which helped out also. Most importantly, I learned that although I prefer a smaller facility, I should not be afraid of a larger facility.

When it comes to interviewing with hospital, visit our website, highwayhypodermics.com and look under "Nursing Info," and then look for "Free Travel Nursing Forms." It is there that you will find a company interview form, and a hospital interview form! Print out a sheet for all your interviews and keep them in a notebook.

Always know the exact location of the hospital. Know what area of town the hospital is in. Then use that information to check out the crime rate of the hospital area.

I might consider working in a higher crime rate area, but I would not want to live there. Do you have a "high crime" plan of action? My husband would definitely be taking me to work and picking me up. I would much prefer to work in an area of low crime, but the amenities of a bigger hospital and town might be worth the 13-week assignment.

For example, I looked at going to a suburb of Los Angeles back in 2004. This was after I had spent 13 weeks in Phoenix. No, I wasn't too thrilled about staying and working in a place like that, but the amenities were the reason I would spend 13 weeks there. I would love to take my son to all the sights around Los Angeles, such as Disneyland and Universal Studios. We didn't end up going because I just wasn't comfortable in having my son in that big of area with a crime rate way over the 200 mark. Now fast forward 10 years, and here I am in the exact same location (Riverside, CA) and having a great time going to the horse races at Santa Anita, spending days off at the beach in San Juan Capistrano, and taking a balloon trip over wine country in Temecula.

What system do I use? I call it my "Glendale" system! While working in Northern Phoenix, I lived in the Glendale area. This was about as much crime as I would ever want to get into. So, when I'm looking at a place to go, I always compare it to the Glendale, Arizona crime rate. Maybe you would want to use your hometown as a measure.

Corporation

How big is the unit will you be working on? How many nurses are on duty? What is the nurse-to-patient ratio? Depending on the number of patient and nurses, the charge nurse is required also to take patients. This affects the amount of time they are going to have to assist you if needed. Do they have licensed vocational/practical nurses and/or certified nursing assistants? It makes a big difference if you are a registered nurse and not only have all of your patients to take care of but you also have to take care of all the intravenous medications of another nurse (as in a RN helping 2 LPNs in California).

Think of unit specific questions also. In the intensive care unit you might want to know the average number of ventilators, how many surgical patients, how many medical patients, or how many cardiac patients are there on a "usual" day.

As an emergency room nurse, I would want to know if nursing or respiratory therapy does the electrocardiograms. I want to know if I have an emergency room tech to assist me with dressings and splints. Am I responsible for my lab draws, or do the lab techs come to the emergency room and draw?

In this technology and information age you will want to know what kind of charting is done. Do they chart on paper or on the computer? Most hospitals have gone to computer charting, but in 2013, I did work for a hospital that still used paper charting!

What type of computer program do they use? Cerner? Epic?

Meditech? Paragon? Do they have care plan problem charting or subjective, objective, assessment, and plan (S.O.A.P.) charting?

What about the medication system? Do they have a computerized system like a Pyxis or Accudose? How do I obtain medications "after hours"? The time it takes for you to get that medication may be a little slower if you have to have the house supervisor get the medication, or if the hospital has a 24-hour pharmacist available.

One of the most important questions to ask is, "How often do the nurses float and what area would you be expected to float to?" Tell them up front if there are any floors that you would not be willing to work on. Be aware also if you are an ICU nurse, the latest trend is for hospitals to hire ICU nurses that can and will float to ALL areas of the hospital. You will not be an ICU nurse, but you will be a FLOAT nurse.

Next you will need to know about meals. This is especially true if you work nights. At the small hospitals, the night shift is usually responsible for bringing their own supper, but in one place where I worked the night shift received their meals free. Plates of food were left in the refrigerator and we just warmed them up in the microwave at break time. At the larger facility I worked at, the cafeteria was open for an hour or two.

The next thing that I can think of to ask would be about special uniforms or the color of uniforms. I worked in one nursing home where the nursing assistants wore colors and the medication nurses wore a different color. The charge nurses could wear colored pants, but we had to always wear white tops, because the elderly associated "white" with a professional nurse.

Next, you might want to ask about the town, although you should have done some homework on the town already. What is the population? Do they have a seasonal fluctuation? In central California, I worked in a small city in which they had a great influx during the harvest season. During that time of the year it was also very difficult to find a place to live.

What is the average temperature for the time that you are going to be there? Do they have four actual temperature ranges and seasons, or just hot, hotter, hell, and whew, I can breathe again! Is it cold, colder, polar bear, and then a few months of defrost? Personally, I'm trying to get this snowbird thing worked out… north in the summer and south in the winter!

What about natural disasters? How many major earthquakes have occurred in the past few years? How many tornadoes or hurricanes? How many times does the creek rise to flood stage? I arrived in Central California the first of November, and during my 13-week contract we had the December 22nd Paso Robles earthquake. Then I had a repeat adventure the first of May 2014 with the 5.1 in Riverside, CA. I landed in Fort Lauderdale on October 23rd and Wilma landed there October 24th. Although I did miss the Tornado near Nashville, TN by a month, and a tornado in Iowa by 75 miles, I'm probably not the best to give advice on diverting away from natural disasters. Oh yeah, and don't ask why Seattle's worst snowstorm ever was when I was on assignment in Puyallup, WA! HA!

Documentation

Out of all the sections that you will read in this book, this is THE MOST IMPORTANT ONE!!! I cannot stress enough to read, read, and then read again this section until you have it down. This could be the difference between a great contract and a disaster!!!

You've talked to the hospital, and now you are ready to head off to your new destination. Your recruiter or the account manager talks to the hospital and the deal is done on their end, but what about the deal on your end?

This is where things get fun. This lovely document, my friend, is called a "contract" or an "agreement." Everything is settled upon verbally, and then the contract is drawn up and sent to you. Your first assignment before you get to your destination is to read the fine print of the document that will dictate what your life will be like for the next 13 weeks.

Negotiations with the recruiter can sometimes be a tedious job, but every detail must be dealt with. Your first indication might be to think, "We discussed everything, and it's in there." NO! I guarantee you that the first time you do that will be the last time that you do that. I have yet to have a contract that I didn't need to add something to.

Sit down in a quiet place and read your contract, word for word and between the lines. If there is any part that you do not agree with, or have questions about, do *not* sign it until those questions have been answered.

If you have a vacation planned, or if you need certain days off, make sure that you get those dates in writing. It has been my experience that if it is not in writing you may have to just live with the consequences. If it *is* in writing, you are guaranteed those days off.

When you open up your new-hire packet you will find several pages of legal jargon that states that you are going to a hospital or facility to work for a certain amount of time for a certain dollar amount. It says that you are going to act like a professional and that the client-hospital and your travel company are going to treat you like a professional.

The employment relationship is the legal arrangement of the contract. As a staff nurse, you were used to being an "at-will" employee, which means that your continued employment was at the discretion of you and the hospital. As a travel nurse, you will become a "contracted at-will employee." Yes, they can still let you go, but as a contracted employee they are obligated to compensate you for breech of contract.

Another type of relationship between nurse, hospital, and agency is called "match-hire," in which the nurse is matched to the hospital, but the nurse is paid directly by the hospital. In this situation, the agency matches you to the hospital. The hospital not only gives you a regular paycheck, but they give the agency a preset dollar amount for your services. Be careful of this situation, because benefits can be very tricky here. The agency can't give you certain benefits because you don't get a regular paycheck from them, and the hospital doesn't give you benefits because you aren't a full-time employee. This situation can cause further confusion between nurse and travel agency when it comes to longevity benefits.

We should all know our professional responsibilities, but because some nurses do not act professionally at all times, those paragraphs have to be added. This part of the contract states that if you cannot show up for your assignment, then you need to call at least two hours before your shift starts. This section also draws the lines of when you, in effect, "voluntarily quit." Although some companies allow for a "lenient" day, most of the time, if you do not show up for the first day, they consider that a voluntary quit. As a protection to the travel company, a clause is added that states that if you act in a careless manner that affects patients or the client hospital, you can and will be turned into the local authorities and state nursing board.

The professional responsibility section is also where you agree to follow the standards set up by The Joint Commission (TJC), the Occupational Health & Safety Organization (OSHA), and the Nurse

Practice Act. This section also includes the fact that you must keep your credentials and licenses that are required for the assignment current. These include documentation that might be needed relating to your nursing qualifications, including ACLS, PALS, TNCC, and State Licenses.

Next you will find your start date, the end date, the facility to which you are assigned, your shift, your on-call time, and your flexibility or floating capabilities. This section might also include whether or not you have guaranteed hours. Make sure that this section is filled out the way you want it! Especially your guaranteed hours and/or the number of days that they can cancel you per contract/per week.

If you do not want to float or do not want to be put on call, then make sure that is put into writing. If you do not feel comfortable floating to a certain floor, like O.B. or O.R., then state that in your contract. When reviewing this section of your contract, you must also be mindful that part of a travel nurse's job is to be flexible. This is *your* contract, and you must protect yourself! It is very important that you discuss this with the nurse manager that interviewed you. If you were interviewed by a computer, then you must request to speak to the manager if you can't float to certain areas or you need time off.

Your travel arrangements and lodging arrangements should be next. Listed here will be your permanent home address and even your temporary address. It will also indicate what is included in your housing arrangements. With some companies you will pay for cable and local phone, most of them will not pay for those extra utilities. But then again, everything is negotiable in this business!

When it comes to your work salary and housing, get everything in writing, and don't ever take anything for granted. If there are days off that you want guaranteed, ask for them in your contract. If you want every weekend on or every weekend off or you're willing to work every other weekend, specify that in your contract if that matters to you. Put it in writing whether you wish to work overtime or not.

If there is to be any deduction in pay related to a missed shift that should also be included. If you are put on call, these deductions should not apply. Make sure that the on-call stipulations are there in the contract.

Included also might be what you are to be paid for a per diem rate. This rate is a fixed rate that is paid to you for food, parking, and other ancillary expenses that you will incur while away from your home state. As of writing this chapter, the maximum allowed by the government is no more than $74 per day. Out of that, they intend you to use $17 for breakfast, $18 for lunch, $34 for supper, and $5 for incidentals. (Meals & Incidentals, 2016) Taxes should be taken out of your hourly rate but not out of your per diem rate.

You cannot get paid unless you turn in your time slips. These time slips are usually faxed to the company that you are contracted with. Some companies have you also mail the original to them, while other companies have you give a copy to the nursing manager. If a company wants certain information on this form, it is also included in this part of the contract.

The last part of the contract might include more legal jargon about benefits, injury on the job, alcohol use, illegal drug use, and the confidentiality clause. All of these important items are included in your contract to protect both you and the company.

In fact, that is the sole purpose of any contract that you have with any company: it is to protect you, the employee, and the company. In this business, verbal agreements mean nothing. Have you ever watched those court shows in the afternoon? *Always,* the judge wants to know if you had it in writing. If it isn't in writing, you just lost.

A nice recruiter may be a pleasure to work with, but just remember that they are working for the money they get from handling your contract just like you are working for the money by being contracted. While a lot of recruiters are nothing more than salespeople, there are some very good and genuine recruiters that are really concerned about you being happy with your assignment.

And You're Off!

After you have picked out the hospital and travel company you need to prepare for the assignment. The company will send you another employee packet with many official forms that need to be filled out: forms required by the Occupational Health and Safety Authority, the Internal Revenue Service, and other miscellaneous company forms.

You then need to make sure that your living arrangements and transportation arrangements are all squared away. The travel company usually makes flight arrangements, but you need to also arrange for your personal items to get there. Can you get everything in three suitcases?

Some things may have to be shipped by UPS or by a moving company. However, having things moved by a moving company can take away a lot of extra money.

Travel nurses are some of the best shoppers at thrift stores! Take only the bare necessities and then go shopping when you get to your new assignment. If you are going to be living at an apartment complex and do not mind used stuff, watch for what is left beside the dumpsters.

Many treasures have been found there. Not that the items are "bad," but when others move from these complexes you would be amazed at what they leave behind. Just like you, others do not want to drag around stuff, so they leave it behind.

On my first assignment my husband and I found a vacuum cleaner and a futon bed. The lady who put them there came out of her apartment just about that time and asked us if we also wanted her television cabinet. Wow! The cabinet turned out to be a corner television cabinet made out of oak, with room for my son's video games below.

After making the thrift store rounds *then* go to a discount store to purchase the rest of your necessities. When you leave, take the important and/or expensive stuff with you as much as possible, sell what you can, take it back to the thrift store for tax credit, or set it back out at the dumpsters for the next traveler.

If you are moving to an extended stay or motel, things are much easier. They usually have pots, pans, and dishes. If not, go back to the thrift store and get a small and a large pot to cook with, and one or two dishes and cups. Do not forget to also get a microwave-safe cooking dish. Before you leave home, make sure that your recruiter or housing supervisor tells you exactly what "furnished" will mean for that assignment.

If you are staying at a hotel or extended stay, a necessity is definitely a slow cooker. They will usually have a microwave already in place at the motel or extended stay. With a microwave and slow cooker, you can have hot meals ready when you come home from work.

If you're dragging or driving your home with you, you do not have as many things to "pack up," but you need to load the RV with the necessities before you add your other wants and needs of comfort. Included in your RV, you do not want to forget your coffee maker and slow cooker. It has also been my experience that we ladies cannot forget a bag—or two, or three—with our craft and sewing items. I have even been to a few travel trailers with sewing machines right next to their computer on the "dining" room table. Scrap-booking materials are also necessary for some travel nurses.

Be sure to pack your necessary nursing documents, such as your last tuberculosis test, your hepatitis C immunization records, and any other immunization records that your company required you to list on the forms that you sent in. Even though you probably sent them a copy, always have them available.

Pack at least copies of your certificates, and carry your nursing license with you at all times. Be prepared to produce any other documents that human resources may ask for.

Be sure to call the place where you are supposed to stay and inquire as to whether all the necessary arrangements have been made. There is nothing worse than getting to a place and having them say, "We weren't expecting you." Make sure that the landlord of the apartment complex knows when you are expected to arrive, and arrange a tentative time to meet with him/her. I cannot stress enough the importance of getting all your housing arrangements guaranteed before you get to your assignment. This is where the great recruiter part comes in! Oh, and do not forget that wonderful recruiter's phone number.

*** References ***

Meals & Incidentals. (2016, July 16). Retrieved from GSA.gov: http://www.gsa.gov/portal/category/100000

Chapter Seven

Questions About Contracts

The first principle of contract negotiations is don't remind them of what you did in the past - tell them what you're going to do in the future.
(Stan Musial)

The travel nursing contract is the piece of paper that has all the rules about the next 13 weeks of your life. This is a very important piece of paper that may take years to fully understand. There are all kinds of situations that can come up in 13 weeks. After reading this chapter you will have a better understanding about what a contract really means and what happens if things don't turn out as planned. These questions are from novice and experienced travelers all over the United States. Hopefully, they can answer your questions for the future!

Is the contract that you sign with your travel agency a different document than the hospital signs with the agency?

Unfortunately, new travelers do not understand that the contract with the travel agency to the hospital is different from the contract between the travel agency to the travel nurse. This should not be a problem unless there are specifics in your contract about the floors that you will work or the days off that you would like that are not communicated in the contract between the agency and the hospital. This is why communication is so important between you and your recruiter. All specifics of a contract should be discussed with your recruiter before the official document is penned.

~*~

I am a travel nursing newbie and don't have a clue about this thing called a bill rate? Don't I get most of the money from the hospital?

Unfortunately, we have to remember that we have a travel company that also has to pay for utilities, marketing, recruiters, and management. This overhead is paid for out of what the hospital pays for you, the healthcare provider. What the hospitals pays to the staffing company is called the bill rate. Out of that "pie" comes the agency expenses and your salary.

After exploring this with several recruiters, it is my understanding that the bigger companies and publically traded companies take anywhere from 20-30% of the bill rate, while smaller companies usually take anywhere from 15-25%; therefore, it is generally better for the nurse to take a job with a smaller to medium company. We also have to look at the fact that larger companies can get discounts on other things that smaller companies are paying a bigger price for (like insurance).

How will you know the bill rate? Well, most likely you won't, because companies really don't want other companies to know what they are exactly offering to their nurses and where all the money is being spent. It is very important for you to know what the average salary for that area is.

The most important thing you have to remember about this bill rate is that there is so much money to supply your needs, and the travel company and recruiter can only give you so much. For the ease of calculations, we will say that the bill rate is $60/hr. Out of this $60, the travel company is going to take an average of 20%, which is $12/hr. This will leave you $48/hr for your recruiter to put into your pay package. After reviewing my contracts going back to 2003, I have discovered that on average the split is 40/60 between taxable and non-taxable, which would be $19.20 taxable and $28.80 for per diems, which is further broken down 40/60 to $17.28 for housing and $11.52 for meals and incidentals. Therefore you weekly wage (36 hours at a 20% taxable rate), would be $44.16/hour or $1589.76/week.

One thing that I might mention here is that if you are thinking about applying for a car, RV, or house loan, the only thing that banks count is your taxable wages; therefore, it might be wise to take a higher taxable rate. Some will take your pay stubs and a statement from your employer about the per diem wages, but not all of them will.

~*~

I'm also a newbie and don't have a clue how to figure out what is the right salary for the area that I'm looking at. This is my first assignment and I'm totally at a loss. I have been quoted $480 for housing, $533 for meals with a taxable rate of $20, this is a 40 hour/week position in the OR in Boston, MA.

At these rates, the split is $25.33 non-taxable and $20 taxable. Using the average taxable rate of 20%, this would end up being $16/hour after taxed and $25.33 non-taxable for a total of $41.33/hour or $1653.20 per week total income.

According to the standard per diems, you are allowed $228.92/day for lodging and $69 for meals and incidentals. (GSA.gov, 2016) That amounts to $20,831.72 ($228.92*7days*13weeks) for 13 weeks of lodging or $44.51/hour with $6279 for 13 weeks of meals and incidentals or $13.42/hour. This means that according to the law, you can take up to $57.93 for non-taxable per diems. In a perfect world, you would be getting the lowest pay for $30/hour wages (Salary.com, 2016), plus $57.93 in per diems for a total of $87.93, but we don't live in a perfect world, we live in one with bill rates!

Now what do we have available? Considering that they are offering $20/hour taxable income, $12/hour for housing, and $13.33 for meals for a total of $45.33, which means that even at the average rate of 20%, their bill rate is approximately $54.40.

Being that Boston is on the coast and beginning nurses make $30/hour, I would really like to see at least $25/hour but would settle for the lowest of $22/hour. Following the 40/60 plan as above, at $22/hour taxable, we should get $33/hour per diems, ($13.20 for meals and $19.80 for housing), but when you add $22+$33, you come up with $55/hour to live in Boston, and they are working with a $54.40 bill rate? Doesn't take a genius to figure out that something isn't right here.

At my calculations, $22 taxable would equal $17.60 after 20% taxes, added to the $33/hour per diems, that would equal a total of $2024/week for a total take home, and they are offering $1653, which is a $371/week difference and an assignment different of $4823, and that is the lowest amount that I would take, take even the median! Again, doesn't take a genius to figure out that something isn't right here.

~*~

What should I demand/ask for as far as my contract is concerned?

Anything that you talked to the nursing manager about needs to be in there! Yes, most contracts are standard, but your recruiter does have the ability to add in a paragraph. If you discussed floors that you are competent to work, vacation hours, or nurse to patient ratios, that all needs to be there.

~*~

I am wary of asking my charge nurses for recommendations before I get a contract, because they would then know I'm looking at leaving, but I don't have anything set in stone yet. Any recommendations on this? How far out do agencies need recommendations before submitting to hospitals?

Yes, you do need to get a reference in writing from your managers/ supervisors. I would tell them that you are thinking about travel nursing, but don't have any set plans. At this time, I would also tell the supervisor that you do not want this request to be of public notice. When you first apply to a travel company, they are going to want the basics of a resume, 2 references, and a skills checklist. So, unfortunately, you cannot be submitted to another hospital without 2 references.

~*~

I verbally agreed to a contract in New York, but there is a new job assignment in Oklahoma that I'm interested in related to the fact that it is near my parents. Just wondering what the penalties are if I cancel my New York contract and go with the Oklahoma contract?

As the old verbiage says, a man's word is good as a bond. You really need to go with your verbal contract unless you have significant factors that will affect the verbal contract. One of the first things you will need to do is to discuss the consequences of you declining the first contract with your recruiter. The biggest problem is going to be if your travel company has already secured housing at the first assignment location. If housing arrangements have already been made you could be responsible for a three-month lease at the new apartment complex. Other than housing responsibilities, it is your choice whether to stand by your commitment or change to another commitment. Just remember that this is greatly frowned upon by the travel industry, and you may have trouble getting a next assignment with them.

~*~

I have signed a contract to start October 27th in California. The day before I started, I got a message from my recruiter that the hospital does not have all the documents that are needed for me to start. Although I, the nurse, have filled out all the paperwork presented to me, I find out that my travel company has not provided the hospital a background check that had been completed in the last month. Since it's not my fault, shouldn't I still get paid for being at the assignment on time?

There are several factors that come in to play here. Do you have guaranteed hours? The first week is known as the orientation week, do you have guaranteed hours and a certain pay rate that affects just that week? Legally, yes, the company needs to pay you, but that is not what usually happens in reality.

First, you need to realize there are two contracts in effect: the contract that the hospital has with the travel company and your contract with the travel company. The hospital and the agency aren't losing any money, except for maybe if you are taking the company housing, then they are not getting paid by the hospital for that week's housing. The only one losing money is you, the traveler!

You are the one who still has to have lodging and meals for that week. For this example, the contracted amount for housing was $700 with $500 for meals and incidentals. Unfortunately in this contract there was no guarantee for orientation week. If you have guaranteed hours for every week, then the travel company, according to what is in writing, is also contracted for the hourly wage. In a perfect world, the travel company would bill the hospital and then you would get paid, but unfortunately, the company is not going to do that; therefore, the company doesn't get paid, and neither will you. Unless…

The best way to handle this is to turn in a time card that has on it "Available" for all 7 days. I would make every attempt to get someone from the hospital to sign this, but your chances aren't too good. Still, turn it in to your recruiter and get the process to rolling.

It has been my experience that the first thing the company is going to do is throw another contract stating that the first one is null and void.

You have fulfilled your end of the deal, you were in California by the start date of October 27th, but the company has not fulfilled their end by paying you for that week. You didn't work any hours and there is no guarantee for hours on the first orientation week; therefore, I would not expect to get paid for that. Did you still have housing and meals to pay for? Yes! Therefore, according to the contract with the travel company they owe you per diem stipends for that first week to a tune of $1200.

What choices do you have at this point? You can take the 2nd contract with the dates postponed for a week, which will void the first contract. You can NOT take the new contract and "fight" for your contracted money from the first one. Or say the heck with it all and find a new contract and new company.

Now, back to reality…the most precious item to a travel company is called a "lead," that is your contact information, and now that they have you working for them, you are more valuable as a traveler. The last thing they want to happen here is lose a nurse. I say that only to say you do have some negotiating power here.

This has actually happened to me twice in my travel career. The first time, we revised the contract to a week later, but I also got $1/hour more for that contract and I ended up extending in which I received an extra $936 for the contracts. Plus, I got to experience my first hurricane! The second time, which is the scenario above, I finally did get my stipends, but they were given to me as a bonus, in which Uncle Sam took his half from what was supposed to be my non-taxable stipends. This also happened to a co-worker of mine, and she turned in her timesheet showing that she was available all those days, and related to the fact that she had guaranteed hours, she was paid in full without question.

The reason why I mention it here is that this is becoming more and more prevalent in today's traveling healthcare world. Yes, I can see the travel company's side in that they can't pay the nurse because they didn't get paid from the hospital, but legally, a nurse's contract is with the company, and I have no control over the hospital/company contract, but I do have control over the contract between company/nurse. The truth of the matter is that until travel nurses and therapists start making these companies pay nothing will ever change. When they start losing money, then they will start charging the hospitals for delayed contracts.

~*~

I wanted September 25th and 26th off to attend the travel nursing conference. My manager scheduled me for the 24th. I work night shift. This will put me ending on the 25th at 7:00 a.m. Therefore, there is no way I can make my flight that leaves on September 24th at 7:00 p.m.

As night shift workers, we have to remember that we are always a day ahead. If you wanted to be at the conference at 8:00 a.m. on the 25th you should have realized that there was no way you could work the night of the 24th. Therefore it is your responsibility to request off starting the 23rd. There are two conclusions in this scenario. Either you are going to have to work something out with the manager, or you will have to attend the conference one day late, which will mean that you will have to reschedule your flight.

~*~

I need an assignment that starts right after the traveler's conference (the first of October). I found one with another travel company and they submitted me. Problem is, my current recruiter saw the job and also submitted me. The pay is the same. I have heard great things about the first company, and I'm really excited about the switch, but on the other hand, I feel loyal to my first travel company; although, I'm not too thrilled about them putting me in for a job that I didn't verbally agree to them submitting me to.

This is a very touchy subject. The biggest question is why did your primary company submit you without your consent? Next we can look at which company is better to go with. You need to take a closer look at the benefits that you are receiving from both companies. You also need to take a look at which recruiter you trust the most. Because that's what it all boils down to: your recruiter can make or break an assignment.

My biggest question here would be why the recruiter automatically submitted you for this assignment. Did you have an agreement with this recruiter that would allow him or her to submit you without your direct verbal okey-dokey?

This is one of the downfalls to having several companies work with you. It has always been my rule of law to have only one primary recruiter with several others working for me if I cannot find an assignment with my primary recruiter. If you are working with several companies, it is imperative that you keep track of which companies have submitted you for what assignments.

In the end, I would go with your original company unless you have a legitimate reason to change companies. The most common legitimate reason would be if the pay rate was extremely higher with the different company.

~*~

When you are finishing one contract about how far in advance do you sign your next?

About four weeks before the end of my contract, I start looking for another. The truth of the matter is hospitals are usually looking for start dates of as soon as possible to up to four weeks out. That is not to say that some assignments can be arranged for a start date further out, but most are between two to six weeks out.

~*~

I signed a contract over a month ago, but just received notification that I needed an up-to-date physical and urine drug screen (UDS). I am on the road and don't have a clue where I can stop and get these things done.

This situation just happened to me in 2013. I was traveling from Iowa to California and they wanted me to stop and get a physical and UDS. My first the action was to inform them that if they could find a place for me to park a 29 ft. RV, I would be more than happy to get their physical and UDS done. It just happened to be that I was stopping in Arizona for a week and my travel company arranged for my tests to be done along the road. If there is any way possible to stop at a place on the road then get the tests done, but if it is not convenient for you continue onto the assignment location and get it done once you get to your assignment location. As the old saying goes, a failure of planning on their part does not constitute an emergency on my part!

~*~

I'm thinking about going out on my own and taking a seasonal contract. Are there any seasonal positions for the winter?

Yes there are plenty of seasonal contracts! The most are in Florida, Texas, Colorado, and Arizona for the winter. Some of them include: Florida: Lee Health System, Baycare Health, Community Hospital, and Physicians Regional in Naples, FL; Health First Hospital, Punta Gorda, Holy Cross in Fort Lauderdale; and Tenet Healthcare in various locations. Texas: Heart Hospital and David's Healthcare in Austin plus Good Shephard of Longview. Colorado: Centura, University of Colorado, and Aspen Valley Hospital. Arizona: Yuma Regional Medical Center and Banner Healthcare.

~*~

Is it normal to do annual competencies for a new assignment???

Unfortunately yes, you end up doing competencies for each new travel hospital and every new travel company if you switch companies. If you stay long enough at the hospital, you may have to also participate in their annual skills day! That is one of the "bad" things about travel nursing.

~*~

To text, or not to text! Should your communications with your travel nursing recruiter be through text, email, phone, or a combination?

I have found that a combination is best. A lot of the time I now communicate with my recruiter through Facebook messaging. That way she knows when I'm up and awake. If there is something urgent, then I will call her and vice versa. When dealing with contracts, I have found that email is best. This way you have a record of every negotiation that you make.

~*~

What happens if I miss a shift? I saw on a forum the other day that a nurse had to pay her company back for a missed day.

This depends on a few things. Did you have an opportunity to make up the day? How many hours do you have in? To complete a contract 100%, you must have been there all your contracted hours. Your contracted hours should be 468 if you work 36 hours a week for 13 weeks. If you are under this amount, then some companies require you to pay them back for the money that they lost on your contracted hours. One company I know charges $18/hour for the hours that you don't work. This also hinges on the factor of whether or not you have taken company housing or the stipend. With the stipend, you just don't get the stipend or your regular hourly rate for the hours that you didn't work.

~*~

Do all contracts come with a 36-hour guarantee? And what about holidays?

Unfortunately, no…not all of them automatically come with a 36-hour guarantee, but that can be negotiated in your contract. This will need to be discussed with your recruiter if the hospital doesn't already have a policy.

Some companies will have exceptions. For example: "Traveler can be called off once every 2 weeks." Banner Health has a policy in which travelers can be called off one day per week. This is more like a 24-hour guarantee. One year in November, I worked 3 days but got paid for 8 days, plus my housing was not affected.

Holidays are also negotiable if the hospital doesn't already have a policy. For instance, the hospital that I'm at now doesn't allow travelers to work the holidays related to the fact that the workers are all union. If they don't have travelers, then they can cancel regular employees and save on the holiday pay rate.

~*~

What are the perks of renewing a contract?

The first perk is that you do not have to do a mountain of paperwork. You already know the staff, which reduces the stress of starting a new assignment, and you don't have to pack up and move again! Other perks that are optional or can be negotiated is in an increase in pay. They don't have to pay you for traveling from point A to point B again, so ask for that cash!

Also, ask yourself if there is going to be a change in the living conditions? If you are in Alaska or Florida, this could be a big deal! In my last renewal, I asked for an "air-conditioning stipend." Therefore, my pay rate has increased a little related to the costs to turn on the a/c in a travel trailer during the summer in Southern California.

~*~

Can I cancel a contract at any time for any reason? What are the penalties to do that?

A lot of this depends on why you are cancelling or quitting a contract early. I had one assignment that was cut 2 weeks short related to the fact my father came down with Guillian Barre Syndrome. Although I was willing to come back and work my two weeks, the hospital wrote down, "11-week contract completed in good standing."

If you have an assignment in which you don't get along with someone and your life is a living hell, that may or may not be a reason to quit an assignment. In 2013, I had an assignment in which the nursing supervisor always found something that I was doing wrong. It came down to the point where she even yelled at me in front of patients in the middle of shift change. Although there were personality conflicts, at no time did I feel like my nursing skills were in question, and I also had the backing of the director of nursing; therefore, I stuck it out until the end.

The closest that I have come to having a dangerous assignment was in Myrtle Beach, SC. In fact, this was the end of my floor career. I was working day shift, and it was busy, but we all pitched in together and it was survivable. I actually renewed my contract and moved to night shift (my personal preferred shift). I didn't realize that I was stepping into hell. Most of the night shift was all new graduates who knew everything. Never in my life have I been told that I'm not needed in the middle of a code, that the new grads could handle it. I had up to eight patients all by myself, and the nursing assistants were all busy helping out the regular staff. Needless to say, as a result of having no help, my back gave out and the last 6 weeks of my contract were cancelled. I worked out a deal with my travel company, paid my own housing, and got lucky with no penalty. This is the difference between a great small/medium company to one of larger ones who would have charged me an arm and leg for everything that went wrong in that contract!

I have never had it happen to me personally, but I know of a hospital where three traveling nurses walked off the job (not while they were doing patient care though). They were not allowed to call the physicians at night; they were asked just to write orders. I can see doing this with things you might have standing orders for—over the counter medications (Milk of Mag, Tylenol, Ibuprofen)—but not for prescription medications. This is an example of a situation in which, if you went in front of the nursing board, you would be practicing way over your level. This would most definitely be putting your license in danger; therefore, I would be contacting my recruiter and my travel company to get me out of there. Once again, a great company would stand beside you and not charge you.

That being said, the biggest thing companies are most concerned with is the 3-month lease that they are liable for. Expect to be charged for this. Some companies will even charge you for their portion of the bill rate that they are missing out on. One company I worked with had a flat fee that if a contract was cancelled, I owed them $3000 in penalties.

Remember also, that everything is negotiable!

Does anyone wait until the last possible moment to sign their contract in case something comes up? If so what do you tell your recruiter that is pestering you?

More and more I'm seeing where companies want you to sign the contract within 24 hours. If you don't know for sure if you are all in on the contract, then you really need to make up your mind before you even interview. This is also true if you have other places that you have been submitted. Some hospitals will wait, but some want an answer that day. During the interview ask when you can expect an answer back from them, and also you need to tell them when you will be answering back, usually within two to three days. Any recruiter who "pushes" you into a job within the first few hours is not a recruiter but a used car salesman. With that being said, your recruiter also expects you to touch base with him/her after the interview, and for you to give them an answer within the next few days. If it's been more than 3 days, yeah, the recruiter is going to start pestering you for a decision. You have to also remember you are not the only one applying for that job.

~*~

I have a month left on my contract, and related to snowbird season being over, they are closing down the ER Hold unit, in which I was contracted for. Now they want me to be a hospital float for the rest of my contract. Can they do this to me?

That's one thing about snowbirds, they always arrive and leave at different times and it's very hard to predict when it is actually going to be over. This is the part that we mentioned in chapter two where a traveler has to be flexible and adaptable. Somewhere in your contract you probably have a phrase that you will float to like units. Unfortunately, you are going to be floated 100% of the time now, related to the fact that there are no patients in your unit. Keep in mind, though, they only need to float you to areas of competence. You could cancel the contract, but chances are you will have to pay a penalty.

~*~

I'm a month into my contract and the hospital is already asking me to stay for a year. Is this usual for a hospital?

If the hospital likes you and you like the hospital and the need is there, then yes, it is very likely that the hospital will want to renew you. Renewing you for up to a year is very rare. I could see this though if the hospital is always short staffed, and they know they are going to need someone still in one year. Most likely the hospital will renew you for another 13 weeks. I've also had contracts renewed for 6 weeks and 8 weeks.

When it comes to being at a hospital for up to a year, you have to remember that once you sign that contract stating that you will be there 365 days your tax home automatically switches to your assignment location; therefore, all your subsides will immediately become taxable. This includes all housing, meals, incidentals, and entertainment monies that you have received.

~*~

The hospital that I'm currently at has three different ICU units (Medical,

Surgical, and Cardiac). I am extending my contract for another 13 weeks, but they want to move me from Surgical ICU to Medical ICU. Can they make me change units?

Hospitals can't make you do anything that you don't want to do! On the other hand, this may be an excellent opportunity for you to broaden your horizons. The biggest question is, "What are the differences between SICU and MICU? Do you feel that you are competent to make the switch?" From what I know about SICU/MICU this type of switch would be very similar. You would be a great fit if you had started out on a medical/surgical type of unit. Then you have a little bit of experience on the surgical side of things.

On the other hand, CCU would be the biggest challenge. You would most definitely have arterial lines, balloon pumps, and a whole different plethora of medications. Once again, I would invite you to take a deep long look at your experience. Do you have telemetry or step-down experience?

Don't let your recruiter push you into an assignment that you aren't qualified for also! When I went from telemetry to step-down in 2004, it was with the encouragement of the recruiter that "You can do anything." Related to a misunderstanding of "taking care of post cardiac cath patients," it landed me in a peculiar situation as I learned the difference between a patient coming back with a sheath that hasn't been pulled and a patient coming back with an angioseal. Oh, I learned how to remove sheaths from helping out the other nurses, but the staff was none too happy that I didn't get post cath patients!

~*~

I have been with "Happy Camper Nurse Staffing" for 5 years and really love them, but "Innovative Travelers" has a job that I really want. I know I can switch, but why do I feel so guilty about switching? What is my recruiter going to think of me?

Longevity with one company is something that travelers usually aspire for, but is rarely attained unless you are with one of the larger companies. If you want the freedom to visit all parts of the United States, then there is a chance that you will have to switch companies at some point in your career.

What you have to learn is that even though we get "attached" to a great recruiter, this is a business, and you have to do what is best for you. A great recruiter will be happy for you even though the assignment didn't come through him/her. Just the fact that you are getting to travel to the place that you really want to be should make the recruiter elated for you! If the recruiter pressures you to stay with him/her and makes you feel guilty for leaving them, that recruiter just sees you as a dollar sign, and unfortunately, you have been "pimped out" for the last 5 years!

~*~

I was talking to a recruiter on Facebook, and they have a job that I really want. I sent "Sandy" a resume, skills checklist, and 2 references for them to submit me to Albuquerque, NM. My now recruiter, "Peter", saw the online post that I was interested in Albuquerque and he submitted me also. As we are talking about opportunities 2 hours later, Peter tells me, "Oh, I saw on Facebook where you were interested in the Albuquerque job, so I submitted you. Whatever Sandy was going to pay you, I will pay you $5 more an hour!"

This is wrong on so many levels! First of all, unless you have given expressed written consent for a recruiter to submit you, then no recruiter should be submitting you to anything without you expressed interest. The ONLY time it is okay is when you have only one recruiter working for you and you have given him/her written permission, usually through email, to submit you. This usually only happens if you have a trusting relationship with your recruiter and you have a hard to find specialty, as in House Supervisor. Related to the fact that I sleep during the day, I don't want to wake up at 10 p.m. and know that a job came up, but now a day has been wasted because I was asleep. So, I will give my recruiter permission to submit me without waking me up. This is a very rare thing to occur though!

Unfortunately, this travel nurse lost out on the Albuquerque assignment related to the fact that she was submitted by two different agencies. This also presented a problem in that she no longer trusted Peter and felt like she was being pimped out, so she had to go through the long process of finding a new travel company and new recruiter.

~*~

This is my second assignment with Great States Staffing and my contract ends in two weeks. I was getting a little nervous about not having a job, so I verbally accepted a high paying contract in South Dakota that starts in 4 weeks. I have just been advised by a recruiter at Favorite Staffing that a job in Hawaii has just come up; therefore, I had them go ahead and send my profile. To my surprise, I just interviewed with the hospital in Hawaii and they want me there in 3 weeks, which is just perfect. Now what do I do?

First of all, as much as you would love to go to Hawaii, I would not have allowed anyone to submit me since I already had agreed to go to South Dakota. On the other hand, related to the fact that it is Hawaii, I can understand why you went for it.

First you need to realize that a verbal agreement is your word. If you have verbally agreed then it is usually just a matter of time that the written contract is signed. Also, if you answered yes to your recruiter in an email, then this can be evidence of a legal and binding written contract.

Truth of the matter is that a company will probably not come after you for any monetary penalties unless the lease has been purchased on your housing in South Dakota. Just remember, that you may be held responsible for any costs that the first company has incurred related to you taking the South Dakota assignment.

On the other hand, you are correct in that you have not signed anything. So, legally there is no signed contract that you can be held accountable for.

The truth of this situation is that you can go ahead and take the Hawaii assignment, but be prepared to pay the price of a being a "DNR" (do not return) from the company who submitted you to South Dakota. This may also affect any references that will be needed from that company.

~*~

I recently signed a contract with a hospital in Virginia. It was on my drive from Texas to Virginia that I got the news that the hospital hired someone else and they were terminating my contract.

In this case, we have to look at both the contract with the hospital to the travel company and the contract between you and the company. You have no idea what the contract with the hospital said, but somewhere there had to be a clause about cancelling a contract.

Your contract with the company probably has a clause in there that you are an "at will" employee. Therefore, your chances of getting payment for the entire contract are probably not going to happen.

In reality the hospital should be liable for all expenses that have occurred by the travel company to get it to that point, but holding them accountable probably isn't going to happen. The company will probably just not use that hospital for contracts any longer.

The chances of you getting what is owed to you for expenses of this assignment is probably not going to happen either. Back to reality, you will probably have to cut your losses and carry on to the next assignment.

Is this fair to the nurse and the travel company? Of course not! But there is little that can be done to "make" the hospital pay for the expenses. This is another reason why it is important for a nurse to have a month's worth of expenses saved up so that you can financially float for a few weeks.

What is going to happen here is that you will return home and the travel company will make every effort to find you a new contract as soon as possible. This again is where the great companies are different than the average companies. A great company would make sure that you made it back home safe and sound. An average company will send you greetings and good luck in making it back home.

The unfortunate thing about this business is that sometimes we have to suck it up and take our losses. Some things are just out of our control.

~*~

My contract with Cedars Sinai ends May 15th, but I'm not on the schedule for the last week. My contract states that I do have a 36-hour guarantee. Is the hospital liable for that last week?

First thing that I would do is discuss this with your nursing manager. I would take your contract to her and ask her to be put on the schedule for the next week. In today's world, I would approach this with an email, that way you would have some kind of written account of the communication between you and the manager.

After you have informed the manager of the mistake, it is the manager's place to add on that extra week. If they do not add an extra week, then according to the contract, yes, you are entitled to 36 hours' worth of pay.

Now the reality of the situation, is the hospital going to actually pay for the extra week? Probably not. On the other hand, your contract is with the travel company and not with the hospital. Therefore, legally, the travel company is liable for the extra weeks' worth of pay related to the written contract.

Will the company pay? Depends on whether or not they are a great company or an average company and on whether they can get payment from the hospital. If you are a great travel nurse and the travel company wants to retain you, then yes, usually they do pay. But, if the hospital doesn't pay them and they are all about the money, chances are you are not going to get paid. Then you will have to make the decision on whether or not you want to go with the same company for your next assignment.

~*~

I was cancelled on Monday. Now it is Friday and I have a girls' night out planned, but the hospital called and wants me to come in. They are stating that I have to come in related to the fact that my contract states that I have to be available for any other shifts in that week.

Unfortunately, this phrase is in many travel nursing contracts. It all has to do with that 36-hour guarantee. The hospital sees it as a need that you must work 3 days a week. If you get called off for one of those days, they expect you to be available for another shift in that week. The travel company wants you to work this shift related to the fact that if you don't work, they don't get paid. Therefore, the reality of the situation is that if you don't go in for the third shift then your 36-hour guarantee is going to be null and void. If you can go in, then I highly recommend it. This lends to your credibility of being adaptable. If you have had a warming up for the party, then absolutely do not go in, but I would not be expecting my 36-hour guarantee either.

~*~

I just received my new contract for my assignment in Arizona. In this contract it states that I will make $20/hour for the first 36 hours of orientation. Huh? Can they really get away with this?

If you sign that contract then yes, they can get away with this! Remember, as a travel nurse it is your first duty to read your contract over with a fine-tooth comb. I would shoot this back to my recruiter and tell them that I did not agree to the ridiculous orientation rate.

Then the ball is in their court. They can talk to the hospital, but ultimately it's their decision on what rate you should be paid. Remember that your contract is with the travel company and not with the hospital.

A contract is a legal and binding agreement between two parties. If you do not agree to the lower rate for orientation, then we do not have an agreement between two parties.

I would really try to work this out with your travel company, but if it means that much to you, then no, you are under no obligation to accept the contract as written, and the whole 13 weeks is out, not just the first week.

~*~

I just accepted an assignment in Texas and after my first week of orientation I'm scared to death. I'm horrified by what I have seen from patient safety issues, to safety of the staff, to putting your nursing license on the line. I'm just not sure that I'm willing to put my life or license on the line, but what is my recourse?

First of all, I totally believe that the only reason to walk out on a contract is when you feel you nursing license is on the line. When it comes down to it, the charge nurse and the director/manager is not going to be with you when you are standing in front of the state nursing board defending your license.

If for any reason you feel that your nursing license is on the line… RUN, and don't look back. Of course, while you are running you will need to notify your recruiter of why you are running. Any great travel company will totally stand by you on this, or you don't need that travel company.

~*~

I was working the telemetry unit and my back "seized" up on me. It felt like someone was tugging on my spinal cord and the pain was extreme. When I went to the ER, they classified it as a repetitious injury. Can I get cancelled from my contract by the hospital if I was injured?

What usually happens in this case is that your contract is cancelled related to a workman's compensation injury. Unfortunately, I know about this first hand. In 2007, the day shift had given a patient Lasix at 6:00 p.m. By the time I came on at 7:00 p.m., the medication was effective and I spent the night getting a patient up and down to use the restroom. By the end of the night, my back as seized up and I couldn't move without severe pain. It was like someone had grabbed my spine and squeezed every time I moved. I ended up in the ER an hour after work. After an MRI, I was diagnosed with a herniated L4/L5, which ended my contract.

Related to the fact that I could no longer work, my contract ended on that day. The only expense to my travel company was my housing. I ended up paying for my housing for the next month and staying in South Carolina for physical therapy.

At any time that you are injured, workman's compensation should take effect. Therefore, the company is liable for any compensation that you are owed. In my case, my travel company was liable for my damages and not the hospital. This is why travel companies have to have workman's compensation insurance on you.

This pretty much ended my career as a telemetry nurse and I had to make the transition back to ER and then to House Supervisor. Every injury is different and depending on the final outcome, you may or may not be able to return to the floor. As for your contract, if you are not able to complete the contract related to an injury then workman's compensation should be liable for the difference. Talk to your travel company! A resolution can be worked out.

No chapter can answer all the questions that a traveling nurse has about contracts, but it is my sincere belief that we have touched on the most common problems that arise in travel nursing. If you have some other situation that you need help with, please don't hesitate to contact me at highwayhypo@yahoo.com.

*** References ***

GSA.gov. (2016, July 20). Retrieved from General Services Administration: http://www.gsa.gov/portal/category/100120

Salary.com. (2016, July 20). Retrieved from Salary Wizard: http://swz.salary.com/salarywizard/Staff-Nurse-RN-Hourly-Salary-Details-Boston-MA.aspx

Chapter Eight

The Nitty Gritty About Taxes

In this world nothing can be said to be certain, except death and taxes. (Benjamin Franklin)

One of the most challenging aspects of traveling will be the tax issues that you will encounter when filing your annual returns and navigating the laws that apply to travel reimbursements. Between 2011 and 2016 there were over 25 healthcare staffing agencies under IRS audit and many others in industries that employ mobile professionals. During this process, many travelers have had their returns examined as a part of the IRS' effort to collect evidence about agency reimbursement/per diem programs. Some agencies under audit have all the personnel files of travelers placed in an accessible area so IRS agents can randomly examine documentation regarding the traveler's tax home status, pay rates, reimbursements, and whether the agency followed their established procedures. Unfortunately, the average recruiter has no idea how the tax laws apply to travel reimbursements and many travelers, who are equally clueless, unknowingly violate the regulations. And of course, there are a fair percentage of travelers that purposely flaunt the rules to their advantage by misrepresenting their tax home status to the staffing agency AND encourage others to do the same. This can be said for any industry but since healthcare staffing compensation involves tax-free reimbursements in a multistate context, the burden of compliance is higher.

Tax Home and Permanent Residence Rules

Why is this so important?

Travel reimbursements, which consist of lodging/housing, meals, and transportation, are excluded from taxable compensation (non-taxable)[1] when you are working temporarily away from your tax residence. The average traveler working a full year of contracts saves between 6 and 9 thousand dollars when they have a legitimate tax residence. If they are keeping a tax home by duplicated expenses of a main home / assignment home, the savings must be offset by the costs of that residence to derive the actual benefit. When you multiply those savings by the number of travelers in all industries, the value of tax revenue that is lost is eye popping. Not to mention, the payroll tax savings the agencies enjoy, as there are no employment taxes assessed on reimbursements as opposed to wages.

The concept of a *tax residence* is difficult for many to grasp as it is often confused with a *permanent residence;* these are two different concepts though they may often be the same place.

Permanent Home, Permanent Residence

A permanent home or a permanent residence is your legal home. It is related to the concept of *domicile*. It is also the place that a person intends to return to after a temporary absence. A permanent residence is primarily determined by the legal ties one has to an area. A driver's license, car registration, voter registration, resident professional practice license and to a lesser degree, church memberships, mailing address, and bank accounts. These connections all point to a permanent residence in a state and, more particularly, a specific community. However, these associations do not constitute a tax residence.

Tax Residence, Tax Home

A tax residence or tax home is one's *Economic Home*, and the tax regulations define a tax home as the principal place of income/business. In other words, it is the general area in which the taxpayer earns the majority of their income on a year-to-year basis. One can

1 The technical term for the tax free stipends, allowances, or per diems is "Reimbursements excluded from taxable income". We will use "tax free" or "non-taxable" for easier understanding.

have a permanent residence in one place and a tax home in another. If they drive 100 miles to a permanent job, then their tax home is the area of the job, not their personal residence. A good example is a professional sports player. If they play for the San Francisco Giants and have their house, spouse, and kids in Atlanta, then their tax home is San Francisco because that is where the majority of the work is performed. When traveling to Atlanta on road games, they are working away from their tax home despite the fact that they sleep in their own bed at their permanent residence. The expenses incurred for travel are still deductible since they are incurred in Atlanta, for business away from the tax residence.

Determining the Tax Residence

Since a tax residence is defined by one's principal place of income/business, determining the location of one's tax home is relatively simple for most people. If they have one permanent job, then that is their tax residence. Where they live is a personal choice regardless of distance traveled to the job site. There are no deductions for simply commuting to a main job regardless of distance. Some people may have two or more concurrent jobs or work seasonally in one place while maintaining a regular job at home. Nothing really changes as far as determining the tax residence. Just follow the money/income. IRS publication 463, pages 2-6 has a general discussion on this and is helpful since it uses examples drawn from tax court cases.

Some travelers actually maintain a job at home or work each year seasonally at another fixed location. This repetitive and frequent income in the same area follows the tax home concept, and when a traveler has this arrangement, the work at home (or seasonal location) becomes their primary place of income. The other locations are treated as travel assignments for tax purposes.

However, over 95% of travelers have no principal place of income. They mobilize from one job to another and do not stay in the same metropolitan area when they take on another assignment. Note the term "mobilize" – travelers are not "moving" as they are working *away from home*. They may extend their assignments, but they generally do not work longer than a year in one area. This is an important distinction and even shows up when travelers are stopped for speeding. If the officer sees out of state license plates and you say that you have "moved," then the officer may issue a citation or a "fix it ticket" requiring you to re-register your car and change your driver's license to the work state. Not a nice way to spend your assignment. To actually fix this, you would need to go before the judge and show them your temporary contract, etc.

The Exception to the Tax Home Rule

For individuals who have NO principal place of income there is an exception to the tax home. Navigating this *exception* can be like working through an ACLS algorithm. A traveler needs to stay within the specific requirements of this exception as their actions can inadvertently put them back under the tax home rule of a main place of income without prospective planning.

The exception works like this: for those that do NOT have a primary place of income, the tax home is allowed to default to the Primary Residence. For this to work, it requires the traveler to satisfy the following criteria:

1) Having substantial expenses maintaining their dwelling at their residence that are *duplicated* when they work away from home on a temporary job. Duplicated in that they incur expenses to maintain their primary residence and have expenses for lodging at the assignment. (Note that this is the purpose of the excluded allowances.)
2) Have not abandoned their traditional place lodging and working – they have family members at the residence or use the residence frequently for lodging.

These two criteria are actually part of a 3 step test that also looks at any income earned at home, but for most travelers, that is not something that is possible.

Expenses keeping a home

Notice that the exception requires expenses to maintain a HOME. A *home* is not a storage unit, a mailing address, where your friends are, etc. It is a home you own or have a mortgage; an apartment you rent; or an alternate arrangement with a friend/family member. If the rent is paid to a related party (family member), then the arrangement must look, smell, and taste like rent and not be a "stick house." A rental arrangement with a family member should consist of rent paid at fair market rental value or a detailed sharing of the expenses with the other adult occupants of the home. It should also be memorialized on a written contract and there should be a financial paper trail to follow. Finally, rent is taxable income so the person you are renting from should consider reporting the income on their taxes unless you are sharing the expenses evenly with other adults. Determining fair market rental value is easily done via classifieds, Craigslist, or some other third party reference.

Abandonment

This is a highly subjective criteria, however there are some important parts of this to grasp. First, a traveler who never returns home despite spending millions to maintain their home has basically abandoned their home. Limited IRS guidance suggests that one should spend at least 30 days or more a year at home, and it doesn't matter whether that is all at once or scattered through the year. The point is, you should return home regularly. Some agencies even require travelers to return home 45 straight days after two years of traveling. That requirement is NOT an IRS rule; it is simply a way in which the agency seeks to stay compliant with the rules. An agency can establish stricter policies than the minimum set forth by the IRS if they wish. They do not have to be copycats of the lowest common denominator.

When a traveler quits their main job, moves a considerable distance from the old area, and then begins to travel, it poses a risk of losing an audit should one ever occur since they have abandoned their original tax home. Once the traveler has left the old place of work, there is nothing established at the new place. For example, say a traveler has worked in Baltimore for the last 3 years at a permanent job, and then moves to their parents in Colombia, Missouri and begins to travel. They have nothing to abandon in Columbia, MO because they have no recent history of work/residence in the area prior to traveling. It does not matter if they pay rent to their parents, rent an apartment, or buy a home. There is nothing established and nothing to abandon. This can be remedied by taking a job in the area of the new home for a short period of time (like a fully taxable, local travel assignment) and establishing an income base.

The Agency Role

Staffing agencies are required to screen a traveler's tax home status before paying tax-free allowances for lodging, meals, and travel. This is often done though a tax home statement or some document in which the traveler is required to attest to their status. Do not confuse the agency requirements with your own obligations before the IRS. An employer has a lower threshold of compliance than the individual traveler, and many travelers have learned the hard way in audits. Just because it's cool with the agency does not mean it clears you with the IRS as they are not reimbursement / tax home police – they are just filters to help maintain the integrity of the tax system. We will see another example of this shortly.

Illustration

To illustrate the exception to the tax home rule, suppose Jane lives in an apartment that she is renting while working in Phoenix. She is traveling to a trauma conference in Denver over a three-night stay. While she is away from home in Denver, she will continue to have a main place of income as she will return to her job. All of her expenses for transit, lodging and meals are deductible OR reimbursable by her employer since she is away from home on business. Their employer may provide a reimbursement or per diem to cover their expenses.

While she is in Denver, she meets a recruiter exhibiting for a travel nursing agency who convinces her to travel. Jane gives up her job but does not relinquish her apartment. She signs a three-month contract and mobilizes to the Denver location. She has the same transit, lodging, and meal expenses, but since she will be changing job sites frequently and does not have a main place of work, her tax home is allowed to be at her residence since she has significantly duplicated expenses of two dwelling units. Her expenses are deductible or reimbursable by the agency. Alternatively, if she gives up her apartment and keeps a job at home (or at another seasonal location) earning significant income there each year and the travel gigs do not take her back to the same location each year, she has a tax residence at the area of the recurring job since that is her main place of income

Let's take this one step further. Suppose Jane gives up her job AND her apartment and then moves into her parents' home in Phoenix before mobilizing to Denver. She does not pay rent. Jane neither has a main job nor a home that she maintains; all she has is a permanent residence in Phoenix, not a tax residence. In this case, ALL reimbursements for transportation, lodging, meals, and even the value of agency provided housing are taxable as wages. The fact that the agency may pay for the housing does not change this; it is wages just diverted to an apartment and taxable.

Limitations on Temporary Jobs

One-Year Rule

A traveler must be working "temporarily" away from their tax home to receive tax-free allowances for lodging, transit, and meals. The term "temporary" is defined as any assignment that does not last longer than one year in the same area. This is a prospective concept. If you have already worked in the same area for 10 months and sign a three-month extension, the moment the new contract is signed, it commits you to 13 months. **From the signing of the extension, the tax home shifts to the work location.**

Short breaks and returns home do NOT restart the clock since there is continuous income in the same area. This is an area where agency policy and a traveler's obligation are different. When approaching one year of service in a particular geographical area, the IRS's internal guidelines require a minimum 7-month break away between two 12 month stints away from the location of the assignment, preferably a 12 month break. Additionally, an administrative ruling treats a seasonal assignment that one returns to annually and earns significant income as a tax residence UNLESS there is income from another fixed location that exceeds the seasonal assignment. Our guideline for clients is to never spend more than 12 out of 24 months in the same area NOR return to the same area three calendar years in a row. The rationale for this is simple–a tax home is one's principal place of income and when maintaining tax residence under the exception to this rule (duplicated expenses), frequent, repetitive engagements in the same area will back you out of the exception and into the rule since you have an identifiable main place of work. Many agencies impose a 30-day, 3 month, or some other break in service rule before allowing a traveler to return to the same area and continue in travel status. An agency can establish such a policy and, so long as it is followed, the IRS will not normally take issue with it, however, the agency is not expected to POLICE your tax status. They are required to establish a "reasonable belief" about your tax home. Whenever in doubt, consulting with a tax professional dealing with mobile professionals is imperative.

50-mile rules and other myths about being away from home

Some agencies toss around a 50 mile rule or some other mileage benchmark to determine if you are far enough away from the assignment to receive tax free allowances for lodging. Unfortunately, there is no such rule. A 50 mile rule only establishes that you drove 50 miles; it does not prove that you actually incurred reimbursable lodging/meal expenses at the assignment. The time tested rule determining *away from home* travel that has been applied in tax court cases is the *rest and sleep* rule. The assignment must be far enough away to require you to get rest or sleep at the assignment location to fulfill your duties AND actually incur lodging expenses. Logically, why should one receive a tax-free lodging allowance without incurring lodging expenses away from home? This is why truckers who sleep in their cab cannot be paid tax-free per diems for lodging. The same rule holds for meals. Everyone needs to eat so an expense is implied; however, to receive a tax-free meal per diem the rest and sleep rule governs this as well.

Why do agencies continue to use a 50 mile rule or something similar? They are attempting to establish a *reasonability* test. Someone who has to drive 50 miles to an assignment is more likely to incur lodging expenses at the assignment than someone who drives only 25 miles. It should be used as a DISQUALIFYER – not a qualifier. It takes no more effort to require the agency to have the traveler attest to an expense for lodging at the assignment than it does to a mileage benchmark. In some cases it has nothing to do with tax; many facilities (hospitals, etc.) refuse to provide premium pay to staff that live within X miles. The rational for this is that current staff would jump ship for the higher pay working as a traveler.

Renting your residence while traveling

If you completely rent your residence to another party, you have converted the home to a business property. It does not matter that the rent only covers the mortgage; it is the use of the home that is in focus. Since you do not live there anymore, it is not your home to occupy. Accordingly, one can partially rent their home keeping a bedroom for themselves or rent it on a vacation basis to a tenant and still keep the dwelling as a tax residence. One can also have family members in the dwelling that share in the expenses. The point is whether you use the home as your place of lodging as outlined under the abandonment rules discussed earlier.

Storage Units

Even though some storage units are gated communities, they, along with vacant land, empty mobile home pads, etc., **are not residences**. Having a storage unit just means you have too much stuff ☺.

RV as a residence

Using an RV as a second residence is a great way to travel; however, you are still obligated to either keeping a job at home OR duplicating the expenses of a main home while away on assignment. A traveler whose only home is an RV and who takes the RV to the assignment is not *away from home*. The home is going with them. As noted above, an empty pad for an RV or mobile home is not a residence. An RV can be a great travel home if the primary dwelling is maintained OR the traveler has a main workplace. Some mail forwarding services that are popular in the RV community erroneously trumpet that a mailing address is all that is needed for tax home failing to distinguish between a permanent residence and a tax residence.

Multi State Tax

While this discussion on tax residence has probably sent you to the ibuprofen, the really pesky task is your state filings. Outside of rare exceptions, you will file a return for your home state and every state that you work in. It does not matter that you did not earn any income in your home state as your domicile/permanent residence state determines where you file your home state return. The mechanics of state tax filings are relatively simple, but it requires planning to avoid traps that are common to travelers, especially those domiciled in high tax states.

Your home state will tax ALL income earned anywhere regardless of where it was earned. The state you work in will also tax the earnings within its borders. Fortunately, to offset any double tax, the home state will credit you for the taxes paid to the work state. If the home state has a higher tax rate than the work state, you will have to make up the difference. If the work state has a higher tax rate that the home state, you will have no additional tax to pay to the home state even though you will still report the income on the home state return.

There are a number of states with no income tax. This does not exempt residents of these states from paying taxes to states that have an income tax and neither does the reverse apply. The states without an income tax are Alaska, Nevada, Washington, South Dakota, Texas, Tennessee, New Hampshire, and Florida. DC cannot tax a non-resident and the Virgin Islands collects tax through an allocation with the IRS; these jurisdictions function like a state without an income tax

There are some exceptions to this rule most of which involve Border States that consider income earned by a border state resident to be treated as if it was earned in their resident state. The other exception is a weird compact between Indiana, Virginia, California, Arizona, and Oregon. Basically, the formula for multistate tax is reversed. The non-resident state gives a credit for taxes paid to the home state on the same income. For example, an Indiana resident that works in California will claim a credit against California tax for the amount paid to Indiana on the same income.

Some states like PA, IN, and OH impose an additional third level tax for municipalities, school districts, cities, or counties. Of these three, the worst two states are OH and IN. When a PA resident pays more tax to the work state than they pay to PA, they are allowed to take the excess credit to the municipal level to offset the local income tax. Not so with OH and IN. The only way to offset OH municipal income taxes and IN county taxes is by working in another area that has a municipal or county tax. As you can tell, OH and IN are not the greatest states to be a resident as a traveler.

Travelers from states with high income tax rates, those from states with municipal income taxes, and those who work in states without an income tax often wind up with large amounts due at tax filing. It is not wise to wait till year-end to pay these taxes. Tax agencies expect a taxpayer to pay at least 90% of their tax obligations as they earn the income, not at year-end. When 90% is not paid, the jurisdiction will impose an "underpayment" penalty or interest just like a credit card late fee charged when a cardholder does not make their monthly payment.

To avoid this, the traveler should make estimated payments through the year to their home state or see if the agency payroll operations can handle a second state of withholding. Agencies are only obligated to report and withhold for the work state, not the travelers home state

Residency Issues

Filing the correct residency status on the tax return is extremely important. A traveler should always file as a resident of their home state and a non-resident in the work state. Many tax preparers and travelers attempting to do their own returns file as part year residents where they work. This creates major problems with nurses holding compact licenses, as a home state filing is required as a part of the renewal process. All tax filings produce paper trails and having random residency filings can create a big headache when the audit cycles start.

All that is needed for states to pursue residency audits is a driver's license, car registration, or professional license. Many mobile professionals get disturbing letters from state tax offices asserting residency tax assessments due to legal ties that were mistakenly established in work states while on assignment in the state. NEVER change your driver's license, car registration, or voter registration. They should all stay at your permanent resident state.

Lastly, most states now cross reference professional practice licenses with tax return filings. About 6 years ago our office contacted all state nursing boards and state revenue agencies asking whether they cross referenced data from each other; almost all said they could and many said they did it as a regular practice. This can trigger some nasty letters when a license is still valid in a state that the traveler no longer works in. California is notorious for pursuing professionals with valid CA licenses that have no income from the state. The typical story is that the traveler receives a letter 2 years after they stopped working in CA and are asked to show a tax return. Instead of just asking, they also assess CA taxes on the income earned that year (pulled from the IRS databases) and threaten action if nothing is done. If the notice is ignored or never reaches the traveler, then a lien will be filed.

Suspension of License

Some states refuse to renew or even suspend a professional license for practitioners that have delinquent tax filings or payments.

Deductions, Per Diems, and Paychecks

The starting point of this discussion begins with the tax home status. If you do not have a qualifying tax home, then everything travel related provided by the agency is taxable. If one does not have a qualifying tax home, the goal is to minimize the tax burden by taking the taxable stipend and finding housing that is cheaper. Otherwise, when the agency supplies the housing, the taxes paid on the value of the housing come out of the rest of the compensation.

For those that have a qualifying tax residence the discussion that follows applies.

Reimbursements

An employer can reimburse for expenses that the employee could otherwise deduct on their tax return. For staffing agencies, travel reimbursements are the largest source of reimbursements. Most contracts are broken down between taxable wages and allowances for housing, meals, and transit. Lodging and meals are often reimbursed on what is known as a "per diem basis." Per diems are very confusing to those that have never encountered them. Basically, per diems are a substitute for receipts. The Federal government maintains a listing of standard allowances for lodging and meals broken down by specific geographic location. These amounts are the maximum that an employer can provide to an employee without an exchange of receipts, so long as the employer has performed their due diligence in screening the employee's tax home status. Since the amounts that are published are a substitute for receipts, the fact that the employee spends less than the allowance is ignored. In other words, you keep the difference between the allowance and what you spend. Sound too good to be true? Talk to any trucker and they will tell you that they find the cheapest accommodations to maximize the value of their lodging per diems.

Expenses in excess of reimbursements

Since the reimbursements you receive are broken down by category, whenever your expenses in a particular category exceed the reimbursement, you have deductible expenses. Lodging is almost always covered under a per diem method and as we mentioned, the excess is not taxed as the per diem provided functions as the receipt. For meals, you can use the Federal per diem rate as your deduction. When the published rate exceeds the meal reimbursement, you can deduct the difference. The same applies to travel pay, and since most travel pay is a capped amount, many travelers have deductible expenses in this category.

Short list of deductions

Travelers can deduct the following assuming the tax home requirements are satisfied: transportation, lodging, and meal expenses *mobilizing to the assignment* less travel pay; expenses for meals, reasonable local business transportation, and lodging *at the assignment* less reimbursements (remember that lodging per diems are their own receipt); and finally, the expenses returning home or *to the next assignment*. There are other costs such as shipping, tolls, etc. that are part of this list as well. A traveler can also deduct trips home during an assignment or between extensions, but these deductions cannot exceed what they would otherwise deduct had they stayed at the assignment location unless they return home to work. One word about reimbursements: if an agency pays a per diem/allowance/stipend and does not specify an allocation between lodging and meals, the payment is deemed to be 60% for lodging and 40% for meals. The reason for this is that meals are only 50% deductible and the employer cannot arbitrarily assign all per diem to lodging. The IRS views per diems as an aggregate of lodging and meals unless the lodging is paid dollar for dollar or provided directly. There has been a trend during the 2014-16 tax years of some agencies paying a ridiculously low meal rate to get around this 50% limitation. In this case the meal rate should be added to the lodging and then the total split 60/40 to keep with the rules.

How agencies construct their pay

When agencies assemble a contract, they always start at the bill rate they receive from the hospital/facility client. The proceeds from this bill rate are then divided between an admin fee (about 20–25%) to cover costs/profit, taxable wages, and reimbursements. This tight matrix creates some of the issues with low wages. When more is paid in reimbursements, taxable wages and/or profit must give etc. Some agency business models seek the lowest taxable wage possible and the highest per diems to make the contract more valuable to the traveler plus save the agency payroll taxes. Some travelers have contracts paying $8–10 an hour as a result. On the other end of the spectrum, there are agencies that concentrate of crisis shifts only providing company housing (or by receipt) and pay a high taxable hourly rate. Then there is the remaining in the middle.

Some travelers mistakenly believe that an agency is bound by the published per diem rates, or even more incredulous, they think that per diem payments come from a mysterious government subsidy for healthcare travelers. As mentioned earlier, per diem rates are the MAXIMUM that an agency can pay without receipts—it is not the standard nor the minimum. An agency can provide anything up to the published rate or nothing at all. Also, per diems are DAILY rates anticipating expenses for hotels. Since a traveler is generally in the area for 13 weeks, a lower rate would be more reasonable.

This is important to note when you are negotiating a contract as tax-free allowances are worth more bottom line than a taxable wage; however, there comes a point when the rate is too low to be acceptable. For the average traveler, a tax free dollar is worth around $1.40 based on a 15% Federal tax bracket, 5% state rate and 7.65% FICA/Medicare tax. This value rises with higher incomes and tax brackets so it can only be determined accurately when using expected income for the year and total tax on that income. A tax-free dollar is worth more because taxes reduce the net take home amount and $1.40 represents what one would have to make before taxes to have $1. This value is a good tool to use when comparing contracts, and since a tax-free dollar varies in value for different wages, consulting with a tax advisor may help make the comparisons more accurate.

Caution on low wages

One may walk away from this discussion thinking that the best contract is one with the lowest taxable wage and the largest per diem; however, the lower the wage, the more risky the terrain. The fact that a professional nurse is getting $12 an hour is not the litmus test of a bad contract or agency, but it certainly draws a lot of attention from the IRS and state labor departments, especially when the agency allows their recruiters wide discretion as to the final wage. To illustrate, say Agency X has 4 nurses working in the same area of the same hospital. Nurse A gets 20 taxable/20 non-taxable, Nurse B gets 15 taxable/25 non-taxable, Nurse C gets 25 taxable/15 non-taxable and Nurse D gets 10 taxable/30 non-taxable (per diems are not paid as wages but we will use this for purposes of illustration). Everyone is being paid $40/hr. All changes in wages are directly proportional or traceable to the change in per diems/reimbursements. The IRS calls this wage recharacterization—the practice of shifting a taxable dollar to a non-taxable reimbursement. Realistically, this goes on behind the scenes prospectively before a contract is presented to the traveler; however, this cannot become the substance of the negotiations where a traveler is offered a choice between a dollar of taxable wages and a dollar of tax-free reimbursements. The IRS views an acceptable wage construct as follows:

1) Taxable Wages + Reimbursements = Total compensation

Looks simple, but reimbursements are paid to offset the costs incurred to carry out an employee's duties—not as a substitute for wages. An agency aggressively pursuing the lowest wages constructs a contract in this manner:

2) Total Compensation – Reimbursements = Taxable Wages (specifically—whatever is left over)

If the IRS sees that an agency has a policy similar to #2, it can apply some massive penalties and restate all the non-taxable amounts to taxable wages, requiring employment taxes from the agency. This is currently happening in some of the audits that we mentioned earlier.

"Tax Advantage" and other nonsense

Though the practice has tapered in the last few years, a number of agencies have marketed the tax free amounts of their compensation as a "tax advantage" program drawing attention to the higher take home pay that is supposedly reaped from the arrangement. The IRS is not ignorant to the practice. In one incident a few years ago, an agency that had never had such a program, announced their new "Tax Advantage" program with a full page ad in a traveler publication, touting the increased take home pay of their plan. This was seen by an IRS attorney in Washington who was responsible for the annual update of the per diem policies. What was done with the copy we can only imagine. We have also seen marketing documents touting an agency's tax advantage program as a way to qualify for needs based education grants, Earned Income Credit, and even a way to dodge child support payments.

The take away from this is that it is not kosher to market higher pay because of higher tax free reimbursements. When a recruiter quotes an "after tax equivalent," they are marketing their reimbursements, not their contract or services. When an agency markets their "tax advantage" program, they are marketing their reimbursement as a wage. The lower the wage the greater the risk. Consider the following: 1) Mortgage applications are generally based on your taxable wage, not reimbursements, 2) car loans are based on taxable wages, 3) a 10K a year mortgage interest payment (reported to the IRS) and 20K of taxable income begs the question of whether another unreported income streams exist, 4) Social Security is based on the highest wage years, and 5) Workers Compensation, Unemployment, and Disability are often based on taxable wages. This is not to say that all agencies are up to mischief as the majority are well-run, stellar players in the industry. As in any group of companies however, there are those with questionable practices just as there are bad apples on every tree.

Missed shift charges

Both traveler and agency are looking for profit and we would be short sighted to think that an agency should just swallow the costs when we fail to fulfill our contract obligations. This is not necessarily a tax issue for the traveler, but it touches the tax free per diems that a traveler receives and has an impact on the agency's tax compliance. In short, the best way this is handled is through a penalty—not by withholding per diems. The numbers arrive at the same destination, but since per diems cannot be paid as wages, the best approach for the agency is to pay the per diem for the week and then apply a missed shift charge. Withholding per diems by hours missed indirectly treats per diems as wages.

Take Aways

Traveling is a great way to see the country, expand your horizons and your career. However, you can count on the fact that your tax filing requirements will be no cakewalk and change dramatically. However, anything rewarding requires work, and the work of traveling is worth it. I traveled as an RT over 20 years ago, and my wife and I are still reaping the benefits of a wonderful 3 years. When in doubt, consult the advice of a tax professional that is knowledgeable in the area of both multistate filings, per diems, and is available during the year to assist you as each opportunity arises. The chain preparation firms have staff that can handle travelers but you have to look hard to find them. With chains, a new client is usually paired up with a new preparer and many only work three months a year. The extra effort, and even expense, will go a long way in helping you avoid mistakes, take advantage of any tax benefits available to you, and protect your license.

~*~

This chapter was authored by contributing author, Joseph C. Smith, RRT, EA MS Tax, of Travel Tax® His experience as an IRS Enrolled Agent and former travel respiratory therapist makes him a valuable asset for travel nursing tax information. Not only does he prepare tax returns, he also holds free seminars all over the United States for traveling professionals. As an Enrolled Agent, he defends the returns that he completes. If you get a letter, just send it to him and he handles the case. If the case does go to tax court, he will refer you to an attorney that works with him. His firm is well known and respected by many individuals and is a leader in the travel medical professional tax world. That, and he is just an all-around nice guy. ☺ Check out his website! www.traveltax.com

Chapter Nine

Politics in Travel Nursing

"Politics is the art of looking for trouble, finding it everywhere, diagnosing it incorrectly and applying the wrong remedies." (Groucho Marx)

Although most of us go into travel nursing to get out of the hospital politics, there are a few things that affect travel nursing in a political fashion. Three of the most recent developments include: The Joint Commission (TJC) accreditation of healthcare staffing agencies, the Nursing Compact, and the National Association of Travel Healthcare Organizations (NATHO). This chapter will explore these new elements of travel nursing and how they will affect your career as a travel nurse.

Joint Commission

It's hard to believe, but it has been 10 years now (August 2006) since The Joint Commission set new standards for healthcare staffing agencies. What does this mean for staffing companies? Standards have been placed on the travel-staffing companies and on travel nurses. The staffing companies will have to clearly define the company leadership hierarchy.

The hierarchy of the travel company will include the administrator, director of nursing services, recruiters, and traveling nurses. The recruiter most likely will have a regional supervisor, an account manager, or a recruiting manager. Also in the mix will be the accountant, payroll supervisor, information systems technician, human resources, and a housing supervisor. The new TJC standards will mean that travelers have to get used to the formal processes, but it will also prevent finger-pointing at travelers and in effect will assist in the protection of the travel nurse's license.

The administrator, nursing director, accountant, or chief financial officer will also be in charge of the development and monitoring of an annual budget. This budget will include costs of certifications, cost of management, costs of the nurses, costs of the benefits, and how that amount compares with the accounts receivable through the hospital bill rate. Where is this going to lead?

With the implementation of TJC certifications, the initial cost of owning a staffing company just increased. This cost is proportionate to national versus regional coverage and the overall size of the company. The cost of TJC certification is determined by the number of branch offices the staffing company is operating. Although the initial cost may be in the thousands of dollars, the efficiencies that certification puts in place increases the effectiveness that keep both hospital and travelers happier in the long run. Staffing companies have found that since the implementation of TJC standards more contracts from hospitals have been offered to the staffing companies; therefore, the jobs available to nurses have increased.

Looking back 10 years, nurses have just rolled with the punches on accepting the requirements that have been put onto us. There are now document companies that will keep your profile and send it to staffing companies, but I still haven't seen a change in a getting a "certificate" that is good for a year, we still are finding ourselves doing "hospital mandated" TJC work and "company mandated" TJC work.

A top priority addressed by TJC certification team is a code of ethics—a code that says the staffing office will take every precaution to provide a work environment that is free of harassment, treats everyone equally, and, in short, treats people like human beings. Respect and ethics have other faces, including sticking with your nurses when the times get tough. Nurses must respect their agencies to be truthful and honest in every situation. Nurses must have ethics and professionalism every day on the job, and the expectations should also be there for the staffing agencies.

Another issue addressed by TJC pertains to getting business through other unfair means, including contract discrepancies, making your travel assignment your permanent assignment, and other conflicts between the hospital and the nurse. TJC now mandates that travelers be protected in their contracts, particularly for professional liability insurance, floating, orientation, and incident or complaint reporting.

Contract discrepancies can include anything from unsuitable housing to pay being contracted as one thing and paid at another rate, and a pay rate that is verbally agreed upon then changed in the written contract.

Conflicts can also occur when a nurse wants to continue on as a permanent staffing member instead of as contracted staff. Some companies put a six-month to one year clause in there that says you cannot go from travel to permanent after a certain period of time. Staffing companies must have a plan to deal with the above situations and any others of the like that come up. When there are problems with the nurse's performance the hospital has a right to terminate that contract, but there is usually a conflict between how much the employee is penalized monetarily for housing and travel. If the employee feels that they were wrongfully terminated, they have the problem of a wrongful contract termination. There must be a plan of action to assist with this conflict, which includes incident reporting that TJC requires from the hospital.

There are always two sides to every story, and conflicts can only be solved through a structured plan and the assistance of mediation if needed. Conflicts and problems do not always occur Monday through Friday, 9:00 a.m. to 5:00 p.m. There must be a twenty-four-hour support telephone line available. The problems that do occur must be promptly solved. The longer the problem lingers, the greater the problem becomes.

Every assignment you will hear from your recruiter or credentialing office, "We need to have all these documents in your file since we are TJC certified." They give you a big long list, but how do you know what is really a TJC rule and what is the hospital/company rule? This all can be found in the Healthcare Staffing Services Performance Measurement Implementation Guide – 2nd Edition. (The Joint Commission, 2016)

The latest edition shows that your personnel file must show the following:

- Verification of a current State License for the state the traveler is practicing in.
- Verification of past work experience, an assessment of clinical skills, OSHA training, HIPAA training, and a current CPR card.
- Verification of minimum health screening, including an annual TB test or documentation of a previous positive.

- Verification of previous employers, reference checks, and a criminal records search.

The first thing that the staffing agency is going to ask for is your nursing license. You will only need to give copies of license that are current. If you have a compact license, make sure that your Travel Company is aware of which state is your primary residential state.

The next big issue is that of quality nursing care. Quality must be assured by skills checklists, orientation skills checked off, and standard safety proficiency. Safety issues are addressed initially with the use of skills checklists, which are completed by the nurse upon application for the position. If a hospital reports that clinically a nurse is not able to perform as stated, then it is the agency's job to work with the nurse to either find different placement or help the nurse to obtain the credentials. These skills checklists must also be updated every year.

Another aspect of TJC standards is the issue of quality assurance and making sure that the credentials and experience correlate to the work history record. For example, if the nurse says that she knows about Swan-Ganz arterial lines, wouldn't it make sense that she must have worked in critical care? Standard safety issues, including blood borne pathogens, fire safety, back safety, and safely getting from the hospital parking lot to your floor and back at the end of your shift are also things that need to be addressed in orientation and yearly educational programs. There are rules now about required yearly continuing education, which will hopefully eliminate repeat paper work at your assignment.

Evaluations from supervisors are also an important tool in safety and quality of care. These evaluations are used to determine if the job is really going as well or as bad as the travel nurse states it is. Then again, we have to remember there are two sides to every story, but usually if things are bad, things are bad on both sides, and conflict mediation may be needed to continue quality nursing care.

TJC standards also involve continuing education. Continuing education, as well as experience, are what make a good nurse even better. Education must also be provided for age specific aspects, patient confidentiality, HIPPA Privacy Compliance, Infection Control, and how to help the patients who have been involved in a domestic abusive situation. This is most often correlated in the orientation process and quality of care issues that were mentioned above. A nurse's skills must be kept up-to-date and new education opportunities taken advantage of in the area of expertise.

When these quality measures become issues, then a staffing company must have an organized approach to improve the nurse's performance. This can be done through educational opportunities and other opportunities for improvement. If required, verbal warnings, written warnings, and termination may be inevitable if these opportunities are not taken advantage of. If there is a conflict between what is stated on paper and what the nurse's performance is, the hospital has the responsibility to report it to the staffing agency. What was the problem? What attempts were made to solve the problem? What was the outcome? What is the percentage of travel nurses that stay with the staffing company? Why did the travel nurse leave the staffing company? Were their problems with the company or just problems related to location or benefits?

All this information provided by the hospital, the nurse, and other information from the staffing company pertaining to the employment of the nurse must be kept in a secure and confidential environment. A plan must be in place in order to maintain confidential information about the hospital that is being staffed also.

Along with all of this goes the process for maintaining continuity of information. The records of each nurse must be safeguarded. The information must be available to the nurse, if needed, for other staffing opportunities. Profiles only need to be submitted upon approval of the nurse. Profiles must not be lost within the system! I had a situation where I was transferring to a different office. One week after I had moved, my file mysteriously disappeared from the office. Was my information in a safe and confidential place?

Excellence in patient care should be the number one goal, and setting the same standards for healthcare agencies that the hospitals have to follow also may be just one more warranted step towards providing greater standards for all involved in the field of temporary staffing.

Wondering if your company is Joint Commission certified? You can go to the Quality Check website at www.qualitycheck.org and find your travel company or any that you are thinking about traveling. You will find minimal data there, but at least they show the records of when the last time the company was audited for quality.

The Nursing Compact

In the year of 2000, Maryland, Texas, Utah, and Wisconsin formed what is known now as the Nursing Compact. These four states were soon followed by many others to form a mutual recognition system. To date there are twenty-four states that are in the Nursing Compact, with three others that have a bill signed by the governor, but which have not been put into effect. For a current list of all compact states, see the National Council of State Boards of Nursing's website at www.ncsbn.org.

For a traveling nurse, this is the best thing since the invention of the mobile phone. This means that as a resident of the state of Idaho, I can travel between twenty-four different states without having to obtain a different license. This is only because my home residence is in a Compact state. If you live in Montana, which is not a Compact state, but have an Idaho license, it is *not* eligible for multi-state recognition. If you go to Texas and state that you are working under your "Idaho Compact License," you are actually practicing in Texas without a license, because your home is in Montana instead of in Idaho.

If you have a multi-state license in one state and you move to another state in the Compact, your first license will no longer be valid. For instance, when I moved my residence from Arizona to Idaho, I received a letter from the State of Arizona stating that my Arizona license had been inactivated due to the fact that I now have a multi-state license in Idaho. If your home state is a Compact state, your license will show "multi-state license" or something to that effect.

Your home state is the place where your house is or where you receive your mail if it's at a relative's house. Although the rules for home state aren't as strict as the tax home rules, I would still have as much supporting information as possible to support your claim of a Compact state being your home state. This might include voter's registration, car registration, driver's license, and mail sent to your address.

Another confusing issue about the Nursing Compact is your state of original licensure. Your state of original licensure has *no* bearing on whether or not your license is a multi-state Compact license. In effect, if I moved my permanent residence to Montana, I would no longer be Compact eligible, even though my original license was granted in Idaho. This is related to the fact that I am no longer a resident of the state of Idaho.

The biggest safety advantage of the Nursing Compact is that nurses whose licenses have been revoked or suspended in one state will automatically have a record through a national database; therefore, making it more difficult for a nurse to get a new license in a different state after being convicted of a crime in another state or any other disciplinary action against their license.

When it comes to legal issues, although you practice under your Compact license, you are still required to practice under the rules of the state in which you are practicing. For example, although I have an Idaho Compact license, I am currently practicing in Tennessee. Therefore, at this time I would be held liable if I did *not* practice under the rules of the Tennessee State Board of Nursing, whereas Idaho State specific rules do not affect me at this time.

Be aware also that if you have a license in a non-Compact state that goes Compact, you will need to notify both boards as to which state is your home state. In other words, I also have an California license where I worked for 4 years just previous to traveling. When and if California ever joins the Nursing Compact, I will need to notify both Idaho and California that Idaho is my state of residence; otherwise I run the risk of my Idaho license being cancelled because I received my California license a few years after my Idaho license. Some states will send you a request for your home state verification, but others will just cancel your oldest license. This has happened to some travelers who had to pay to get their legal home state licenses reinstated. It is imperative that you keep each state board of nursing informed of your permanent address at all times for this reason.

Update 2016! A new press release that was received on 07/07/2016. "Missouri has joined Arizona, Florida, Idaho, New Hampshire, South Dakota, Oklahoma, Tennessee, Virginia and Wyoming as a member of the Enhanced NLC."

This will allow nurses to have mobility across state borders, the enhanced NLC increases access to care while maintaining public protection. The enhanced NLC, which is an updated version of the current NLC, allows for registered nurses (RNs) and licensed practical/vocational nurses (LPN/VNs) to have one multistate license, with the ability to practice in both their home state and other NLC states. The enhanced NLC will come into effect the sooner of 26 states passing the enhanced NLC legislation or Dec. 31, 2018. All states, including those participating in the existing NLC, must introduce legislation in the coming years to enter into the enhanced NLC.

"The enhanced Nurse Licensure Compact will include background checks and prompt reporting of information, plus timelier sharing of information among member states. This helps facilitate the state's responsibility to protect the public health and safety of Missouri citizens. In addition, it will decrease redundancy in the consideration and issuance of nurse licenses," commented Rep. Kathryn Swan, sponsor of the Bill in the House. Sen. Jay Wasson sponsored the Bill in the Senate.

Patient safety being of paramount importance led to the addition of new features found in the provisions of the legislation of the enhanced NLC. Licensing standards are aligned in enhanced NLC states so all nurses applying for a multistate license are required to meet the same standards, which include a federal and state criminal background check that will be conducted for all applicants applying for multistate licensure.

The enhanced NLC enables nurses to provide telehealth nursing services to patients located across the country without having to obtain additional licenses. In the event of a disaster, nurses from multiple states can easily respond to supply vital services. Additionally, almost every nurse, including primary care nurses, case managers, transport nurses, school and hospice nurses, among many others, needs to routinely cross state boundaries to provide the public with access to nursing services, and a multistate license facilitates this process. (Kappel, Dawn M., 2016)

I have attempted to answer the basic questions about the Nursing Licensing Compact. If you have further questions, it is always best to call the state board. If you work in a state that is Compact and your license is not a multi-state license, this will not only affect your license in that state, but *every* nursing license that you have. Ignorance is *not* bliss this time.

~*~

The National Association of Travel Healthcare Organizations

In 2008 a new non-profit association of travel healthcare firms was formed to promote ethical business practices in the healthcare travel industry. It benchmarks the new gold standard for behavior that is aligned among member agencies on behalf of travel candidates and clients.

The organization functions to educate the healthcare industry on the benefits of travel healthcare staffing, establishes a set of service standards among travel healthcare companies, shares resources among member organizations, offers formal dispute resolution process between NATHO member firms through an arbitration committee, and assists members in cultivating market growth.

NATHO members are held to a strict code of ethics that was developed specifically for the travel healthcare industry. It is important for travel healthcare professionals and healthcare facilities to keep this in mind when selecting a company to provide services.

NATHO membership allows healthcare staffing firms to access information unique to the travel healthcare industry to include insurance and risk management resources, public relations, shared marketing resources, federal and state legislative issues, ethics and arbitration guidelines, credentialing standards, standards of practice, industry benchmarking, industry statistics, and group purchasing.

Membership criteria includes Joint Commission certification, proof of insurance (professional liability, general liability, and workers compensation), and a payment of the minimum membership fee of $1,000 annually.

The Code of Ethics states that the members are responsible for maintaining and promoting an ethical practice. The Code of Ethics will serve to clarify the manner in which each member of the organization may fulfill its responsibilities to the general public, to clients, to candidates, to other recruitment organizations, and to other travel healthcare organizations. If a dispute occurs between members, the first obligation is for the members to resolve the issue among themselves. It is understood that disputes between members will then go to the Ethics Committee or Arbitration Committee (if it is a dispute over a fee) for resolution.

The ethical rules state that a travel company shall fulfill all agreements made with the hospital and shall not make promises that the travel company believes they cannot keep in full. The travel company has to represent the nurse as accurately as possible with the nurse's employment history and qualifications. The travel company cannot send a profile to a hospital if he or she does not have the approval of the traveling nurse. If a travel nurse's file is submitted by one or more travel companies, the travel company that receives the job offer from the hospital will be honored as the company representing the nurse, regardless of the timing of submittals. If a hospital makes an offer to more than one member, the traveler will choose the company to represent them.

The travel company must provide services that remain in compliance of any applicable law, including complying with federal, state, and local laws governing hiring practices. A travel company must adhere to the credentialing standards established by the Joint Commission.

The travel company shall not knowingly make a false statement about a job opportunity to include responsibilities, compensation, hours, and other pertinent information concerning prospective opportunities. A travel company cannot knowingly deceive a traveling nurse or encourage a nurse to breach a current obligation or future contact. The travel nurse is not allowed to switch companies, but must remain at the same hospital without a 90-day break.

During an investigation by the Ethics Committee, the travel company shall fully cooperate with the Committee or Board of Directors concerning violation of the Code in a timely manner. The two travel companies with the conflict must inform NATHO Headquarters that they have made an attempt to solve the matter between themselves.

In their use of advertising and marketing, they must not make a false or misleading statement about the healthcare staffing company or the services. They cannot publish material misrepresenting the spirit of the Code of Ethics, and they cannot publish something that would make the statement misleading. The travel company cannot compare other company's services to theirs when the facts cannot be factually substantiated. A member must ensure that the jobs they advertise are factual and available.

The staffing company should never discredit the reputation of another competitor, and they must honor agreements between other members of NATHO. They must refrain from defaming, maligning, or falsely accusing another member or competing firm. They also must refrain from intentionally misrepresenting another member to a prospective candidate, client, or another staffing agency.

The Code of Ethics also demands that all staffing company representatives act professionally and in a businesslike manner, not engage in a deceptive or misleading manner, and they must honor both oral and written agreements made with other members. It must never engage in activity that brings dishonor to the healthcare staffing industry.

In accordance with the ethics policy, all staffing companies must abide by strict accounting and taxation standards as set forth by the Internal Revenue Service. It is also understood that violating accounting and taxation laws to gain a competitive advantage is not only an issue of unfair competition, but also puts the client hospitals and travelers in serious risk of sanctions for violating labor laws and regulations. They perform proper use of the non-taxable per diems or lodging, meals, and incidentals allowances or reimbursements. They must also use appropriate classification of the temporary healthcare employees as non-exempt and W2 employees with proper withholding of all taxes, including state income taxes. They must abide by all overtime laws.

The NATHO Ethics Committee will field all complaints to the president and the Ethics Committee. The Ethics Committee will consist of the chairperson and a minimum of three other members. The chairperson is appointed by the President of NATHO for a three-year term. All of the members shall be individuals employed by active member organizations of NATHO and appointed by the Ethics Committee chairperson with the board of directors approval for a three-year term. The chairperson and committee members may succeed themselves. The Ethics Committee shall be responsible for reviewing and acting upon reported violations of the NATHO Code of Ethics or may, on its own initiative, institute an investigation of apparent violations.

In February 2010, NATHO formed a technology committee to assist in the development of software standards for healthcare staffing agencies to share data with vendor management services. The aim of this committee is to provide staffing firms with a database in which venders can enter job order information and firms can match up travel nurses with the information entered from their application profile. At this time, staffing companies have to enter the candidate's information into each vender management system for each job that comes up. By integrating the system, the candidate's information will not have to be entered into the system repetitiously.

Most recently, NATHO sponsored KPMG to conduct a hospital labor cost study to compare the salary and benefits cost of hourly full-time employees in comparison to a temporary traveling nurse. According to their press release on June 8, 2011, the all-in cost of a full-time direct care hospital registered nurse (RN) is on average $98,000/year ($45/hour), of which only $55,739 is base wages ($25.84/hour). Fully-loaded payroll, which includes base wages, employer taxes, and paid time-off represents 76–78% of the total cost of the RN labor force at facilities. The balance comes from non-productivity costs (12–13%), insurance costs (8–9%), recruiting costs (1–2%), and other costs (1%). In other words, the actual cost per hour for a full-time nurse is on average 176% of their base hourly wage. These are important factors in evaluating whether to add staff, increase overtime, or use contingent nurses to meet patient needs.

There are also significant additional "hidden" nursing labor costs, which are mainly the result of non-productive labor hours and associated opportunity costs, as well as attrition and time required to fill a permanent direct care RN position, the KPMG study reports. Non-productive labor hours on average represent 13% of total hours, according to respondents.

Two-thirds of the hospital executives responding to the survey say they are currently using travel or per diem nurses. The key reasons for using traveling nurses were supply-and-demand and the quality of these nurses. These appear to be even more important decision factors than cost. Some of the reasons given, which enable some hospitals not to use traveling staff, include the use of extra full-time staff, part-time employed staff, incentives to limit turnover, and to encourage working overtime, as well as the current economic downturn leading to limited turnover. Many of these factors may be of a temporary nature and increase costs and turnover over the long term. Respondents also stated that the ideal balance is 90% permanent staff and 10% supplemental labor.

Two other studies that are in the beginning stages include a study on the use of the PBDS testing, which is used to evaluate the "competency" of a traveling nurse, and a study on travel nurses who switch companies, but do not switch hospitals.

The study is to determine if the PBDS (Performance Based Diagnostic System) test is being used suitably for traveling nurses. If the test is found to be inappropriate, then NATHO will encourage those hospitals using the test to get rid of it or use it more appropriately.

They are also studying a way to prevent travelers from going from Travel Agency A to Travel Agency B while still working at the same hospital. While there are times when nurses have a genuine reason for switching companies, there are many more who switch companies for trivial reasons.

This chapter is only the tip of the iceberg. NATHO offers so much more with articles of interest for traveling nurses, agencies, and hospitals. These articles include up-to-date news on the nursing shortage, mandated staffing ratios, the economics of travel nursing, travel tax answers, how to choose a reputable agency, how to be professional while on the job, landing the best assignments, and many other tips for the traveling healthcare professional.

All in all, NATHO is making every attempt to create a positive image for the traveling healthcare industry by developing a peer review process that is based on excellence, honesty, and fairness between travel healthcare agencies. This, in turn, will provide better quality service to hospitals, traveling nurses, and ultimately patients.

**Mission, ethics, and standards of practice information were acquired from the website and press releases of the National Association of Travel Healthcare Organization used by permission. This chapter has been reviewed and approved by former NATHO president, Mark Stagen. For more information, please check out their website at www.natho.org.*

*** References ***

Kappel, Dawn M. (2016, July 07). *Enhanced Nursing License Compact.* Retrieved from National Council of State Boards of Nursing: https://www.ncsbn.org/9642.htm

The Joint Commission. (2016, July 20). Retrieved from Health Care Staffing Services: https://www.jointcommission.org/hcss_certification_program_performance_measurement_implementation_guide_2nd_edition/

Chapter Ten

Testing In Nursing

"I think that probably the most important thing about our education was that it taught us to question even those things we thought we knew. To say you've got to inquire, you've got to be testing your knowledge all the time in order to be more effective in what you're doing." (Thabo Mbeki)

Tests, tests, tests… you thought the NCLEX was the last test that you would have to take in nursing, but it was actually just the beginning. When you decide to make travel nursing your career, you just locked yourself into nurse testing up to four times a year.

Unfortunately, there are some tests that will be required for each hospital that you go to. I'm warning you now, your company will have you fill out all those tests and competencies before you get to your hospital in Paradise, and don't be surprised if you have to fill out all that information again on the hospital's forms or computer system.

Basic Company Testing

There are some tests that are required by the travel company that you will have to take before ever landing a travel assignment. These are tests that are required usually by regulatory agencies once you get to the hospital (Joint Commission, Medicaid, and Medicare).

Mandatory tests that you can expect to take include HIPAA, age specific knowledge, hazardous chemicals, fire safety, newborn safety, infection control, drug use in the workplace, ethics, environmental safety, fall prevention, biological terrorism, patient rights, body mechanics, restraints, prevention of medical errors, cultural diversity, disaster preparedness, sexual harassment, violence in the workplace, and violence in domestic situations.

Not only will you have to fill out a skills checklist for your specific specialty, but most of the time, you will also have to take some kind of computer testing for your specialty before you are even submitted to a hospital. Some of these checklists and tests include general registered nursing, progressive care, NICU, PICU, telemetry, medical, surgical, intensive care, dialysis, psychiatric, and emergency room. Other added tests may include pharmacology, basic rhythms, and intravenous therapy.

Performance Based Development System

This is a wonderful test that was developed by Dr. Dorothy delBueno in an effort to test a nurse's critical thinking, interpersonal relation, and technical skills. The test consists of several short videos that are played in which the nurse is required to recognize the problem, assess what interventions need to take place, what he or she would expect the physician to order, prioritize how and when those interventions are to take place, while also taking into consideration conflict resolution, customer satisfaction, team building, safety in performance, and use of equipment.

The travel nurse will be required to take the test that most closely corresponds to that of their specialty. To date, testing is provided for adult Med/Surg, critical care, OR, OB, mental health, and ER. In the hospitals that I have researched, those whose specialty is pediatrics, rehab, or telemetry, are required to take the Med/Surg test. Those whose specialty is step-down, surgical intensive care, medical intensive care, coronary intensive care, or neurological intensive care are all required to take the critical care test.

Here is where the first problem lies: there is no test developed for every nursing field that exists. If I'm hired for telemetry and take the Med/Surg test, how does that prove my competency for the telemetry floor? If I'm hired for rehab and I take the Med/Surg test, how does that prove my competency for things such as how to manage the care of a patient who is trying to walk again versus a patient who is having an acute stroke? Some hospitals just give everyone the Med/Surg test as a "basic" nursing test, even though the nurse has been in the Psychiatric or OB field for ten years. Therefore, if they are going to use this for a competency-based assessment, they need to have it for the specialty that we say we are competent in and have been practicing in.

When you take this test, you will be shown about a twenty second video of a patient who is having some kind of an acute distress, and you are supposed to figure out what is going on with that patient, what you should do first, and then progress from there until the patient is stable.

Here lays the second problem in the fact that you are expected to write every little thing down that you can think of to do. You also have to come up with a diagnosis that you think the physician is going to assign to the patient. Remember, you have to do all this after viewing just once a short video, approximately 20 seconds worth. Since when are nurses trained to diagnose what is wrong with the patient? Do you take notes or watch the video? I would think it is very difficult to accomplish both at the same time.

There is also a section that concentrates on prioritizing in "must do," "should do," or "could do." If a patient has a potassium level of 6.2 and another patient has a troponin level of 0.144 with a CKMB of 4.5, which is going to be my priority? Although the potassium level may cause some cardiac arrhythmias and would be considered a "should report," the elevated troponin and CKMB levels are more important and a "*must* report," related to the fact that they are indicative of a myocardial infarction.

These tests require you to write down not only what you would do in step-by-step format but also why you are doing those things. One of the catches here is that you must write down all the little things. For example, for an elevated potassium level you would not only notify the physician, who will probably order Kaexylate, but don't forget to also write down that you would hold the morning and evening doses of potassium.

To help study for this test, think about some of the situations that you have been in that require prioritization. What would you do or say if the charge nurse asked you to do orientation of a new nurse, but you have a really busy day and all of your patients have different procedures to go to on which you might have to accompany them? What would you say when a nurse comes up to you and asks you about another nurse, and what would you do if you witnessed a nurse yelling at a patient in the room?

Diseases that you might want to be familiar with and write out a care plan to study include heparin drips, insulin drips, diabetic coma, stroke, acute myocardial infarction, chest pain, increased intracranial pressure, digoxin toxicity, pneumothorax, congestive heart failure, chronic obstructive pulmonary disease, pulmonary embolism, renal failure, hemorrhage, pylonephritis, bladder retention, ilieus, thrombocytopenia, peritonitis, pain control, and sepsis.

What effect does this test have on travel nursing, and why is it so controversial? It is because the test was designed to assess a nurse's strengths and weaknesses for an orientation process that is tailored to that nurse, but what the hospitals are now doing is using the test to "weed out" travel nurses that are "incompetent." This includes several nurses that have been "practicing incompetency" for twenty years. Excuse me? The state board of nursing says that I have been competent to practice nursing for twenty years, but a 20-second test says that I'm a danger to my patients?

I have heard numerous stories where the first week of orientation was going great, the hospital really liked the nurse, the nurse's professionalism and competence was being proved daily with everyday situations, and then their contract was cancelled because all of a sudden some test says that they are incompetent. Now she has no job, but she still has a three-month lease on an apartment.

Let's just say that I have accepted a job in Naples, FL (several hospitals there are known for using the PBDS testing for travelers). To date, the average apartment lease is $1200/month plus a $600 deposit, and I will have to lease the apartment for 3 months in order to move in. This will be at a cost of $4200. After I lease the apartment, then I have to drive there from my home in Idaho. At the current rate of $0.54 for the 2600 miles, this would make my travel expenses $1400. At a rate of 500 miles per day, it will take me approximately 5.23 days to get from Idaho to Florida, which will mean 5 nights in motels at an average of $100/night for a total of $500. Then we will need to add $50/day for food, for a total of $250. That would mean my total for the trip and the three-month lease, not including rental furniture that will need to be returned, will be $6350.

My question now is, what nurse in his or her right mind would take a $6300 gamble on a test that is not being used as it was originally designed?

Unfortunately, there are some nurses who do take this gamble, and that is why the hospitals continue to use this testing system. I don't have a problem with a testing system to prove competency, but it needs to be arranged before a nurse drives across country only to have her contract cancelled. I don't even have a problem with the PBDS test, as long as it is being used to see where nurses are lacking and orientation is customized around what the nurses are lacking in. Travelers are expected to receive very minimal orientation and hit the floor running; therefore, extended customized orientation is not an option.

Basic Knowledge Assessment Tool

The BKAT is a Basic Knowledge Assessment Tool used to test a nurse, usually in an orientation setting. According to the author's design, it is not to be used as a "weeding-out tool" for hiring purposes. It was designed to validate the knowledge of nurses who have previous experience in medical/surgical nursing, pediatric and adult intensive care, adult and pediatric emergency care, and telemetry nursing. Clinical specialists and educational coordinators are to review the tests and gear educational in-services to those questions that nurses have missed.

The tests were originally created by Jean Toth, PhD, RN, MSN, CV-CNS, BCCC, from the Catholic University in Washington, DC, over thirty years ago. It was created by using analysis of literature, clinical proficiency, and a panel of master degree level nurses who excel in their specialty. The test can be copied, but it cannot be altered in any way.

It is an educational tool that, according to the author, Jean Toth, is to be used for determining the educational requirements of nurses. There are BKAT's for ER, Peds, etc. The author states in her preamble to the "test" that it is *not* to be used for hiring or firing.

According to nurses who have taken the test, the questions are very similar to those found on the NCLEX exam. It is a very practical exam and tests your knowledge of every-day situations. The questions are very basic, should be relatively easy to an experienced nurse, and should be very passable for even a new graduate.

The medical/surgical BKAT is an eighty-eight question test that measures the knowledge of nurses in the areas of cardiovascular, endocrine, renal, neurology, gastrointestinal, pulmonary, and wound care, along with a few questions on pain control, fall prevention, infection control, communication, spiritual care, emotional care, drug calculations, advance directives, blood transfusions, hypothermia, and obesity. This test takes about forty minutes to complete.

The Adult ICU-BKAT is a ninety question test of critical care nursing knowledge of cardiovascular, pulmonary, monitoring lines, neurology, endocrine, renal, gastrointestinal systems, along with a few questions on infection control, hypothermia, burns, and spiritual care. The test takes approximately forty minutes to complete.

The telemetry/progressive care BKAT evaluates the nurse's knowledge of cardiovascular, neurology, endocrine, renal, pulmonary, gastrointestinal/parenteral items, along with a few questions concerning infection control, hypothermia, monitoring lines, and emotional/spiritual care. There are eighty questions that take approximately forty minutes to complete.

The pediatric BKAT is a ninety-six question test that tests the nurse's knowledge about pediatric cardiovascular, monitoring lines, pulmonary, neurology, endocrinology, renal, gastrointestinal, and other areas, including play therapy, drug overdoses, and family-centered care. This test takes approximately forty minutes to complete.

The Neonatal ICU-BKAT is a seventy-five question test that evaluates the knowledge of the NICU nurse. The questions cover cardiovascular, pulmonary, gastrointestinal/parenteral, neurology, renal, monitoring lines/catheters, family/spiritual care, with a few questions on developmental care, sleep, pain, and blood incompatibilities. This test takes approximately forty-five minutes to complete.

The ER-BKAT is a one hundred question test that determines the basic knowledge of the critical care nursing aspects in the Emergency Department. Items on the test include: cardiovascular, pulmonary, neurology, endocrine, renal, gastrointestinal/parenteral, OB/GYN, pediatrics, with a few questions on drug abuse, trauma, psychiatric situations, rape, and mass casualties. It takes approximately forty-five minutes to complete.

The Pediatric ER-BKAT is an eighty-question test that assesses the basic knowledge in pediatric emergency care. The content measures the knowledge of the nurse in cardiovascular, neurology, pulmonary, trauma, endocrinology, gastrointestinal, renal, and miscellaneous items to include drug abuse, sepsis, and psychiatric situations. It also includes a question about blood transfusions, burns, child's play, conscious sedation, drowning, immunization, mass casualty, and obesity. This test takes about forty minutes to complete.

A copy of the test can be obtained by sending $15.00 and the agreement form to Jean Toth, PhD, RN, MSN, CV-CNS, BCCC, BKAT

For Critical Care Nursing, PO Box 6295, Washington, DC 20015. Nurse staffing agencies are not allowed to request the tests—only nurses who are subject to taking the test. More information and the agreement form can be found at www.bkat-toth.org

Chapter Eleven

Preparing For an Adverse Reaction

"There is nothing as strong or safe in an emergency of life as the simple truth."
(Charles Dickens)

With each travel assignment we prepare for the adventure, live the escapade, and then our journey ends, only to perpetuate us on to the next quest. But along our path, we cross over many bridges in the form of emergencies, troubled waters, and even the end of the road.

These things are more difficult to face as travelers related to the fact that we are out there on our own and don't have a community or family right there to surround us with comforting thoughts. However, a determined travel nurse doesn't give up; we just pack up and move on down the highway of destiny.

Emergencies Along The Road

In case of a medical emergency we are taught to dial 911, but whom do you call when you are hundreds of miles away from home? Be prepared! Be very prepared!

The first line of defense in case of an emergency is to have an emergency planned for. Not that we really want one to happen, but we don't want one to happen and get caught, as they say, "with our pants down." We certainly don't want to panic.

The first order of business is to have someone to call, like AAA, Good Sam's Emergency Road Service, or OnStar®. Keep those numbers, usually found on your membership card, in your wallet, above the sun visor, or in your purse. Other important phone numbers to have with you include your recruiter, you bank's number, your car insurance agent's number, and a network of friends along the way.

A network of friends is not only handy to have as a safety feature, but could also be a convenience feature. I have several friends around the country with whom I have worked before that I keep track of and have even had a few invites for supper and a place to stay. I wouldn't recommend staying with someone whom you have only met online, but I would definitely stay with someone that I had worked with before.

If you have not invested in a good nationwide cell phone, now is the time. For years I refused to get one because I had a C.B. and it was free. Although very handy at times, some people just aren't comfortable with a C.B. When I was driving forty miles every day to work, the C.B. was all that I had. The few times that I had problems, I would holler at the trucks to send a policeman or highway patrol.

Have a friend or relative lined up to call every time you stop for gas. I always call my parents along the way so if something does happen to me they have some idea where to start a search. Of course, you would also want to let that person know what route you are taking.

Although taking some cash is a good idea, taking too much is not a good idea. Keeping a national ATM card, with access via a pin number, is a must. I carry no more than a hundred dollars cash and attempt to pay for everything off my debit card, which comes out of my bank account. This also gives me documentation for the tax man.

Before embarking on that next adventure, it is also a necessity to visit your local mechanic to get the oil changed and the fluids checked, along with tire pressure. In the trunk of your vehicle you should keep extra food, blankets, and water, in the event that you have a roadside emergency.

Make sure that you have a good map or a great GPS. The best maps with nationwide truck stops can be found at the major "chain" truck stops, and some even provide a list of rest areas. If you are traveling in an RV there is also a map put out by Good Sam Rand McNally Road Atlas. This is a great map that not only finds all the tourist traps but also gas stations for RVers. Another great resource is the location of tourist information centers as you go into a state. They not only provide you with free maps, but they also have interesting facts about the territory you are about to travel through. GPS is a great tool! In fact, as a traveling nurse, I won't have a vehicle without one. There are some really good portable ones out there on the market, and even cell phones have them.

When on a long trip and you haven't ever been that direction, you should always start looking for a gas station when you reach one-half of a tank. By doing this, you don't risk getting too low before finding a place to stop. This is especially essential if you are pulling a travel trailer or traveling in a big motorhome. It is also important to remember that your gas mileage is a lot different when you are pulling a trailer. I always reset the gas mileage counter when we are pulling the trailer so that when it says, "You have 100 miles to empty," I know that that is going to be fairly accurate with pulling a trailer.

When getting out of your vehicle to fill up with gas or go to use the restroom, always be aware of your surroundings. If someone makes you feel uncomfortable, stay in your vehicle and travel to the next rest area if possible. If you are a female traveling alone, it is not advisable to drive at night, although I do know some women who aren't afraid of traveling alone because their safety is ensured by Smith and Wesson.

That brings up the point that, if you do have a concealed weapon, be sure that you know the concealed weapon laws in the states you travel through. Other personal safety items to keep in the vehicle consist of a large flashlight, which not only provides light but can be used as a weapon. They also make a small light that goes on your key chain with an ultraviolet light that will blind someone, giving you time to get out of a dangerous situation.

Another great tip is to carry a device in your glove compartment that will allow you to break the glass or cut your seatbelt in case of a traffic accident. And last but not least for on the road, always make sure that your spare tire actually has air in it! You won't be too happy if you find this out along the Interstate.

In the good ole days when I started traveling, we always found the phone book and the yellow pages to help us locate the nearest urgent care center, grocery stores, laundromat, and emergency vet. Now-a-days, all you need is a smart phone! Yelp! Is based on the yellow pages and is a great resource when first getting to your new assignment.

For financial safety it is always best to have at least a month's worth of income saved up before you head out on the road. I know, this is impossible for some travelers, but please keep in mind that contracts can be cancelled without too much notice. Also, in case of a major mechanical failure during your travels it is nice to have a financial cushion to pay for repairs.

By using these tips and others, you can travel from state to state with peace of mind. By preparing for an emergency, you will know that if something does come up you won't be the first to hit the panic button because you will have everything under control.

Surviving The Assignment

My patient is screaming down the hallway about how it is time for his pain shot; the nursing supervisor just called and my admit will be here in ten minutes; when I called the surgeon about his patient that is bleeding through his dressing, I got yelled at because I didn't call sooner; and if the patient in room 19 doesn't quit hitting at the staff, then I'm going to have to call his doctor to get an order for restraints; and, of course, there is no one to help me because I'm the traveler making "all the big bucks." Are travel nurses supposed to think that this is "normal" behavior, or is this nursing abuse?

Pain management is getting to be a bigger and bigger issue. Yes, there are patients who have legitimate pain management needs, but how many patients are we taking care of where this is their second admission this month because they need their Dilaudid or Fentanyl fix? This is a bigger issue in the emergency room than I see on the medical-surgical floor. The 1-10 "oucher" scale was supposed to help this, but some patients have figured that out and will rate their pain as a 15.

What are nurses to do about the abuse of the system? We just have to continue to assess our patients in a timely manner and provide them with their medications as ordered by their physician. There is nothing that we can do about this abuse of the system because we are not that patient and we have been told that we have "no right" to judge how much pain a patient is really in.

Working with physicians that are verbally humiliating, degrading, and have a total lack of respect for us as professional nurses is also a fact in the life of a nurse. In a recent study published by the Association of OR Nurses, over 90% of nurses that were polled were subject to verbal abuse by a physician. Is that true just in the operating room? I don't think so! Try calling certain physicians in the middle of the night.

What can we do about verbal abuse? What usually happens is that we vent to a few of our co-workers, we keep the patient in mind, and go on and do our job to the best of our abilities. Remember, the patient is why we are there. We must call that physician in the middle of the night to protect our patient, as well as for protection of our license. Yes, it is sad but true, a lot of the things that we do are to "CYA"...

Abuse of a nurse by the patient is also a common problem that nurses face during the work day/night. The patient is under the influence of narcotics, illicit drugs, or alcohol and we're supposed to be understanding because they *are* ill. Would they still be ill if they weren't under the influence of all those substances?

We must protect our own health, and when a patient gets violent we need to seek assistance as soon as possible. If we are injured, this needs to be reported to the nursing supervisor as soon as possible, along with getting medical treatment for ourselves.

Do we have the right to press charges against that patient for assault? In some states, a hospital employee definitely has the right to press charges against that patient. There should be no difference if that patient injured us inside the hospital or if he injured us out on the street. If nurses get hurt, who is going to take care of us?

Of course we have to deal with all these things, plus "crises" that occur, and not make any mistakes on these hectic floors. Time management is the key to survival! Come out on the floor, check out your patients, and then get a routine going. No, you can't stick by your routine every day. Things happen—patients have surgery, patients have to be admitted—but if you have your routine set up, then it is easier to accomplish these other tasks without getting overwhelmed.

When an overwhelming situation comes along, ask for help. Hostility may be amongst the nursing tribe because you are a travel nurse "making all the big bucks," but you can't do everything by yourself. You need to ask for help. If you can't get anyone to help you, approach the charge nurse and then work your way up the chain of command, from Charge Nurse to House Supervisor to Manager to Director of Nurses. And of course, always notify your recruiter of what is going on first. They will be your first line of defense.

Travel nurses are in hospitals all around the United States and select foreign countries. They are there to help. They are not going to these different places to be abused by other staff and patients. You should be flexible in helping your co-workers, but you don't have to take severe abuse. Keep on working hard, and remember that you only have thirteen weeks there.

Don't be afraid to stand up for yourself. If you become overwhelmed with the pressures to the point that your license is in danger, you must get out of the contract. I will repeat again, if you become so overwhelmed that you are putting your license in danger, you must discuss this with your recruiter about your option to get out of the contract and out of the hostile environment.

You were looking for a job when you found that one. Life may have its speed bumps, but just keep on trucking down on the travel-nursing road. The next assignment has to be better!

Looking back at all the tough assignments that I have had, I asked myself, "What are some of the techniques that I use when things are getting tough?" As we all know, travel nursing isn't always fun. We have plenty of good times and adventure, but there are also times when we want to run and hide.

Yes, survival is what it is all about. It's a jungle out there, and a travel nurse must be prepared to tread through the trenches and come out a victor! Come on, there can't be much difference between surviving in a jungle and surviving a terrible nursing assignment. Here are my eight tips for survival in Travel Nursing:

- Shield yourself with a "net" by putting a smile on your face. How can you be sad if you are smiling? Sure, you might be smiling only on the outside, but that is a start. You can shield your patients from knowing that you are having a bad day by wearing a smile!
- Get rid of the leeches! Stay away from the people who are most commonly the causes of the frustration. Sometimes you can't ignore them, but by getting more involved in nursing care and farther away from the nurses' station, these leeches will bother you less.
- Delve into the trenches. One of the best diversion tactics that I rely on is to spend more time with my patients. Take time out just to visit with them. What can you do for your patients instead of sitting up at the nurses' station, listening to what all is wrong with the unit?
- When the rainfall is heavy, find shelter. You need to have someone that you can talk to. If nothing else, call your recruiter or get online and find a travel nurse support group. Sometimes things will resolve themselves if you just tell your frustrations to someone who is going to give you a little reassurance.

- In a violent storm or monsoon season, it may be necessary to find a lifeboat. Talk to your recruiter about what is going on. Talk to the unit manager or someone who is over the person that you are having trouble with. If you really feel like your nursing license is in danger, go talk to your recruiter and/or an attorney about getting out of your contract.
- Finding the light in the midst of darkness. Find something that makes you happy and surround yourself with it. Go on a little shopping trip and get something that you have always wanted. Find a place of serenity and immerse yourself in meditation. On bad days I tend to come back to my little "ole'" RV, sit outside, and watch the waterfall that I have in my pond. I would definitely suggest that a travel nurse have some kind of small water feature to travel with her.
- A positive attitude can keep some of the mosquitoes from getting to you. Go into each day with the thought that you are going to make it the best that you can. That may change twenty minutes into your day, but at least you started out on the right foot.
- Count down the days. Seeing the light at the end of the tunnel is always refreshing. Mark on your calendar the number of weeks left, or even the number of shifts left. Twenty-seven days sounds a lot better than two months!

These tips and tricks may not work for everyone; but for me, they keep me going through tough assignments. Remember that you are there because of your love for nursing, without all the politics. Remember that you do care, and that there will always be the next assignment and another exciting adventure in travel nursing.

Using Laughter To Survive Your Assignment

We've all heard the saying, "Laughter is the best medicine," but just how can it help you through your day as a traveling nurse?

Our first two weeks at a new assignment have to be the toughest. It is at this time that I am trying to adjust to my new surroundings, and I want to make a great first impression that I really do know what I am doing.

During the first weeks, you have to SHOW them that you know

what you are doing, you just can't tell them what you are good at doing. It is only after establishing that professional relationship that I start mixing in a little humor.

A little humor can go a long ways in making an assignment the best that it can be. Even with my worst assignment, humor is what made my day worth getting up for. Not humor with the other staff members, but humor with my patients. Even though the staff was under a lot of stress and anxiety, my patients were well taken care of and smiling because I was busy taking care of them with a little bit of everyday humor.

On the second day that I have a patient I can usually gain a smile by asking, "Can I listen to see if your heart is beating today?"

This simple attempt at humor will give me a feel about how well the patient is going to accept humor. With some patients that is the start of a wonderful humor relationship, and with others they let me know right quick that they are not in the mood for my little antics.

Some of my most memorable patients haven't been those that are grumpy, but those patients that I have laughed with through their many days at the hospital. Not only does this elevate my patient's mood, but it also has been proven to make a difference in muscle relaxation, neuropeptide release that affects depression, vasodilatation that reduces hypertension, and it also has the most effect on the hardening of attitudes.

Many of the places I have been want me to extend, not only because I'm there to work and do my job, but because of the humor and positive attitude that I bring to the unit.

Someone was fumbling with the foil surrounding a suppository the other day and I just calmly walked over and asked, "You know why they include the directions to take off the foil… because you *know* that someone did *not*." That little chuckle took away some of the stress that she was having opening that silly packaging.

You don't have to be a comedian to be a humorist. Just keep your eyes open to everyday occurrences. Did you ever wonder why they put the instructions on the hemorrhoid cream, "Do not take PO"? Yes! Because someone, somewhere, was eating the hemorrhoid cream and complaining to the company that it wasn't helping their hemorrhoids, and that they couldn't eat anything larger than a jellybean. And whatever possessed the hospital to contract "Seymour Butts" to design hospital gowns?

Now that you're smiling…take that smile to work and make your co-workers and patients smile right along with you.

Unexpected Contract Termination

What is a nurse to do? What constitutes valid grounds for the nurse to break a contract? What constitutes valid grounds for the travel company to break a contract?

A travel nursing contract is a legally binding contract and cannot be broken for just any old petty reason. Part of the nursing shortage problem can be from working conditions and unsafe living conditions. Unsafe living conditions can include housing that is inhumane or insecure.

As a travel nurse, you need to do your homework on your accommodations before signing the contract. By using www.apartments.com or www.homefair.com, apartment and general housing location's crime rates can be checked out. What crime rate is an acceptable crime rate for you?

Is the hospital located in the inner city with prostitutes and drug dealers walking the streets at all hours of the night? Do not hesitate to call security to escort you to your vehicle if you decide to take a job in a higher crime area.

The biggest problems usually arise with the larger companies that place corporate politics over taking care of their nursing staff. Recruiters can only do so much for their nurses in a larger cooperation. If the problem does not get solved, give them written notice as to why you believe that the contract has been breached, and that you are terminating your contract due to their breach of contract and their inability to resolve the problem.

Serious health problems, such as orthopedic and/or medical problems that require surgical interventions, motor vehicle accidents, or medical problems that will take an extended period of time to recover (e.g. hepatitis) are legitimate reasons to end a contract. If you are not able to complete your contract because of health reasons, the request to terminate the contract early must be in written form, which also needs to be accompanied by a physician's statement.

Health reasons for immediate family are also considered a legitimate reason to ask for early termination of a contract. In 2004, I had this happen to me when my father came down with Guillian

Barre Syndrome. I was lucky enough to be on week 11 of a 13-week contract. The manager asked me when my last day was, and put on my records that I completed my contract on that day in good standing. Now, that being said, my company was very good also in letting me out of my contract two weeks early, but this will not always happen! The company can make an attempt to collect housing costs for the days that are left on the lease.

I don't know of any travel nurse who can say that they have never been homesick at some time in their travel-nursing career. Keep your ears and eyes open for other travel nurses at work. There are more and more local groups on Facebook where traveling healthcare professionals can meet up, such as the Southern California, Northern California, and Pacific Northwest travelers groups.

Chapter Twelve

Traveling as an LPN

"Nurses may not be angels, but they are the next best thing." (unknown)

Long before I was a registered nurse I practiced as a licensed "practical" nurse. Although I never traveled as an LPN, I remember hearing all the time, "If only you had your RN license." At the time, I was doing just fine as an LPN. I never had a problem finding a job, I made more money than I did as a nursing assistant, and still had the satisfaction of assisting the elderly.

That was twenty-four years ago, and I still don't think things have changed that much for LPNs. You still have LPNs who are happy to be just who they are and who don't want the added stresses of being a registered nurse. To tell you the truth, there are some days when I wish that I was "only" an LPN. I still believe that the LPN is a great asset to the nursing community.

With all that being said, the real question comes to this: how does being an LPN affect you as a traveling nurse? Should LPNs be able to travel? Of course. I've met a lot of them that I would much rather work with than some RNs, but there are some hospitals that are phasing them out. This may elevate the degree of difficulty in finding a travel nursing job, but it *does not* make it impossible. To explore this option for LPNs, I asked for now traveling LPNs to answer a few questions. The following is what I found out.

When asked if they felt like LPNs were being phased out, most believe that no, they were not, and that LPNs should be able to travel as well as RNs because nurses are needed everywhere. The real trick is to gain a lot of experience and have a willingness to travel to limited areas. One nurse stated, "Being an LPN is a financial move; it covers the bases and as in any structured situation, the higher you get the less scutt work you wish to do. Oddly, many good LPN's don't see things the same way. Nursing is about getting away from the bedside, and that is understandable; it can be a horrible place to be, but an LPN knows she/he will always be there, so they take it much more to heart than the "office nurse," and they are always the last in line for respect. It's a sad way to make a living."

At the time of writing this chapter it seems like Core Medical Group, Medical Staffing Solutions, LLC, and Supplemental have the most jobs. I would suggest that you find two or three companies and always keep your file updated so you can be ready to go when there is a job that comes up.

When it comes to reimbursements, the jury is split 50/50. Half of the nurses told me that their compensation was no different than an RNs, and half of the nurses stated that their compensation was a little less. From this I gather that it all depends on what company you travel with. Your travel pay, including your housing stipend, meals and incidentals, should be the same whether you're an LPN or an RN. The thing that will be different, as usual, is your regular hourly rate.

When it comes to education, the travel companies do not seem to supply much more than your BLS/ACLS. A few hospitals have offered nurses staff positions in trade for financial reimbursement for additional schooling to get their RN license. Personally, I went to school for my RN through the University of the State of New York/Regents/Excelsior program while practicing as an LPN instead of having a hospital pay my tuition in trade for two years of service. That is a great option if you really want to further your education, but you do not have to get your RN to be a great travel nurse. Be aware though, that California currently does not accept new applications from Excelsior Educated nurses.

Most LPNs struggle with finding good assignments and the lies, misrepresentation, lack of respect, and lack of recognition. Other facts that challenge LPNs are reimbursement issues, and they believe that facilities do not want to put their money on LPN's.

Some of the rewards of traveling as an LPN include meeting new people, receiving more pay, traveling to places that are happy to see you, and the occasional recognition. Other LPNs stated that serving the healthcare community and seeing areas of the United Stated that they have never previously visited is what makes it all worth the while to them.

According to most of the company websites that I visited you must have at least two years of experience, with at least six months of recent hospital experience, and LPNs in a hospital setting must be IV certified. As with traveling RNs, you will still have to file a work history, background check, mandatory education (Blood borne pathogens, OSHA, Fire, HIPPA, etc…), and your skills checklist.

When it comes down to finding a nursing job, I would try one of the companies listed below to find a job. I have personally tested these companies out and they do have jobs!

~*~

LPN/LVN Travel Companies

Accountable Healthcare Staffing – A place where they actually LISTEN to what their nurses want and need. Their recruiters are all very experienced and educated. They are here to find you the best possible package out there. AHCStaff.com

Advantage Medical Professionals – Super-charge your nurse job search with Advantage Medical Professionals! We're a Healthcare Staffing Agency dedicated to offering best nursing jobs in the US. www.advantagemedicalprofessionals.com

Aureus Medical Group – Their mission is to "be the staffing provider and employer of choice by helping people and companies achieve their goals." www.aureusmedical.com

Cirrus Medical Staffing – At Cirrus Medical Staffing, they specialize in the placement of traveling medical professionals. If you're ready to earn top dollar, leverage your skills and enjoy the adventure of a lifetime, this is where your journey begins. www.cirrusmedicalstaffing.com

Convergence Medical Staffing – All of their recruiters are experienced with travel healthcare professional placement. When they tell you something, you can take it to the bank. If they are wrong, they admit it and if a mistake were to occur related to your contract, they eat it. cmstaff.com

Core Medical Group – Their highly experienced staff works with the country's best hospitals to obtain new LPN jobs daily. www.coremedicalgroup.com

Fusion Medical Staffing – Fusion Medical Staffing places both nursing and allied staff nationwide. They are a small privately owned company who makes personal service a top priority. www.fusionmedstaff.com

Health Providers Choice – HPC is a mid-sized private owned company which offers Registered Nurses (RNs) travel, local contract, and per-diem positions. www.hpcnursing.com

Medical Solutions – They offer opportunities for RNs ranging from staff RN to LPN and allied health. Their jobs are located all over the 50 states. www.medicalsolutions.com

Premier Healthcare Staffing – Apart from all of the outstanding service standards that you can expect, Premier Healthcare Professionals will never be beaten on a pay or benefits package. www.travelphp.com

Primetime Healthcare – They make a difference related to their industry knowledge, true competitive pay, and additional bonuses for contests throughout the year. www.primetimehealthcare.com

Randstad Healthcare – At Randstad, they work hard to know their candidates. They also work hard to know their clients in effort to make a better match between the two. www.randstadhealthcare.com

Traveling as an LPN may be a little more difficult than traveling as a RN, but it *is not* impossible.

Chapter Thirteen

Allied Health Traveling

"The best therapy is actually the more aggressive kind when they break you open; they unleash you." (Cara Delevingne)

Physical Therapy

Physical therapy is a very rewarding occupation in which you can take an immobile patient and have him up and walking in a relatively short time. As a traveling physical therapist you can travel to acute rehabs, home health, pediatric centers, skilled nursing facilities, sub-acute facilities, and wound care clinics.

Many states now require physical therapists to have a master's degree, and it would be a good idea to have at least two years of experience before hitting the road on a travel assignment.

PhysicalTherapyJobServices.com is a full-service informational website that allows physical therapists easy access to many essential resources when planning for a change in your career path. www.physicaltherapyjobservices.com

Occupational Therapy

When soldiers from WWI came home they needed help to get back to doing even simple everyday activities of daily living. Their "occupation" was getting back to a normal everyday life as best as they could. To help accomplish this, specially trained people called "occupational therapists" were trained to help them get back to the simple tasks of combing their hair, putting on their boots, and feeding themselves.

Occupational therapy has come a long ways since then. Not only can you now help those who need assistance at home, on the job, or in school, but you can do that for several types of people in several locations around the United States.

In order to be a traveling occupational therapist you will need to be certified in occupational therapy and have at least two years worth of experience at a hospital or rehabilitation facility.

Speech Therapy

A speech pathologist doesn't just deal with how well you speak, what dialect you speak, or mispronounced words; they are much more than that. They find themselves working in acute care, long-term care, and rehabilitation facilities with those patients who are having problems eating and swallowing. Others also work with patients in improving their linguistics, communication, language disorders, phonetics, and language development.

After completing a "swallow evaluation," speech therapists will make a recommendation on what type of food the patient can handle, whether it is whole, cut, soft, ground, or pureed. A speech pathologist or therapists may also accompany a patient to radiology for a barium-swallow evaluation.

Respiratory Therapy

According to the Department of Labor, faster-than-average employment growth is projected for respiratory therapists. Job opportunities should be very good, especially for respiratory therapists with cardiopulmonary care skills or experience working with infants.

The employment of respiratory therapists is expected to grow 19% from 2006 to 2016, faster than the average for all occupations. The increasing demand will come from substantial growth in the middle-aged and elderly population—a development that will heighten the incidence of cardiopulmonary disease. Growth in demand also will result from the expanding role of respiratory therapists in case management, disease prevention, emergency care, and the early detection of pulmonary disorders.

Older Americans suffer most from respiratory ailments and cardiopulmonary diseases such as pneumonia, chronic bronchitis, emphysema, and heart disease. As their numbers increase, the need for respiratory therapists is expected to increase as well. In addition, advances in inhalable medications and in the treatment of lung transplant patients, heart attack, accident victims, and premature infants (many of whom are dependent on a ventilator during part of their treatment) will increase the demand for the services of respiratory care practitioners.

Job Prospects

Job opportunities are expected to be very good. The vast majority of job openings will continue to be in hospitals; however, a growing number of openings are expected to be outside of hospitals, especially in home health care services, offices of physicians or other health practitioners, consumer-goods rental firms, or in the employment services industry as a temporary worker in various settings.

Respiratory therapy travel is one field that is gaining in popularity; therefore, the field of traveling respiratory therapy is also growing at an astronomical rate.

For All Therapies

Once you have the license and experience you can travel to hospitals, assisted-living facilities, rehab centers, long-term care centers, outpatient clinics, and home health agencies.

Therapists receive some of the same benefits as a traveling nurse including housing, meals, incidentals, continuing education, free health, dental, and vision insurance along with some short-term, long-term, and life insurance.

~*~

Allied Health Placement Companies

Accountable Healthcare Staffing – A place where they actually LISTEN to what their nurses want and need. Their recruiters are all very experienced and educated. They are here to find you the best possible package out there. AHCStaff.com

Cirrus Medical Staffing – At Cirrus Medical Staffing they specialize in the placement of traveling medical professionals. If you're ready to earn top dollar, leverage your skills, and enjoy the adventure of a lifetime, this is where your journey begins. www.cirrusmedicalstaffing.com

Convergence Medical Staffing – All of their recruiters are experienced with travel healthcare professional placement. When they tell you something, you can take it to the bank. If they are wrong, they admit it and if a mistake were to occur related to your contract, they eat it. cmstaff.com

Core Medical Group – Travel Nursing Jobs. Whether you are seeking a travel nurse, permanent nursing job, or seeking an allied health job, they've got hundreds of health care jobs to choose from. www.coremedicalgroup.com

Fusion Medical Staffing – Fusion Medical Staffing places both nursing and allied staff nationwide. They are a small privately owned company who makes personal service a top priority. www.fusionmedstaff.com

Flexcare Medical Staffing – Flexcare specializes in contracting Registered Nurses, with at least one year of current experience, in acute care facilities throughout the nation. www.flexcarestaff.com

Health Providers Choice – HPC is a mid-sized private owned company which offers Registered Nurses (RNs) travel, local contract, and per-diem positions. www.hpcnursing.com

Host Healthcare – Host Healthcare is dedicated to going "above and beyond" to make each assignment memorable. Combined with the other benefits that they offer, they believe that they have the best all-around package for their therapists. www.hosthealthcare.com

IPI Travel – IPI Travel excels in the Travel Nurse, Allied and Rehab Industry providing quality healthcare clinicians in all 50 states. Their network of relationships, with top healthcare facilities across the country, will open doors for you where other Travel Companies fall short. www.ipitravel.com

Medical Solutions – They offer opportunities for RNs ranging from staff RN to LPN and allied health. Their jobs are located all over the 50 states. www.medicalsolutions.com

Premier Healthcare Staffing – Apart from all of the outstanding service standards that you can expect, Premier Healthcare Professionals will never be beaten on a pay or benefits package. www.travelphp.com

TotalMed Staffing – TotalMed prides themselves on genuine relationships and currently walks in their travelers to each assignment if it is at a new client and local. www.totalmedstaffing.com

Trustaff – Placing healthcare professionals in travel nurse jobs, pharmacy jobs, therapy jobs, and more. www.trustaff.com

Chapter Fourteen

Traveling When You're From A Foreign Country

The greatest obstacle to international understanding is the barrier of language. (Christopher Dawson)

Just because you were not born in the United States does not mean that you cannot become a traveling nurse in the United States. It does take a while to get your work visa, take language tests, take a registered nurse competency test, and make the voyage to the United States, but it is a worthwhile journey when you think about all of the new adventures you will be experiencing. Being a traveling nurse once you have at least one year of experience will give you an excellent way to travel around the United States and see all the wonderful sites. This chapter was written to help you accomplish that dream.

Finding a Nursing Job In United States

With the nursing shortage getting bigger and bigger every day, finding a nursing job in the United States is easier than ever. Nurses who are from the Philippines, Canada, Australia, or England can easily gain employment in the United States by following this simple guide.

With the help of CGFNS (The Commission on Graduates of Foreign Nursing School), nurses' qualifications are acknowledged, confirmed, and proven in reference to the education, registration, and licensure of nurses worldwide. Through this commission you will need to finalize a Visa Assessment and Work Screen.

In the Work Visa Screen, an educational investigation and evaluation of the foreign nursing license is conducted. Nurses are also required to pass the NCLEX or the CGFNS International Qualifying Examination and an English Language test, such as the TOEFL or IELTS.

One of the first requirements is getting an associate's or bachelor's degree in nursing and then passing the NCLEX (National Council Licensure Examination), which is a computer nursing competency test.

In some states, if you did not go to an English-speaking school, you will have to take the TOEFL (Test Of English as a Foreign Language) before you can receive your license as a Registered Nurse. This is the most widely used test for workers from a foreign country.

Some states are starting to use the IELTS (International English Language Testing System). It is a language test that measures the ability to communicate in English in listening, reading, writing, and speaking.

After passing the NCLEX, a language test, and obtaining a Visa Screen Certificate you are qualified to submit an application for a nursing license in the state where you reside. Then the fun begins in finding a nursing job.

You would be surprised how many travel companies now welcome foreign educated nurses with open arms. Some of the companies that will assist you include Parallon, Assignment America, Global Healthcare Group, Health Careers of America, Nurse Immigration Services, Pacific Link Healthcare, PPR Healthcare, Preferred Healthcare Staffing, Premier Healthcare Professionals, and Worldwide Resource Network.

Coming to work in the United States can be a longer process than you would like, but it is important to keep your eye on the cloud with the silver lining ahead of you. Someday, *it will* all be worth it!

CGFNS

The Commission on Graduate of Foreign Nursing, also known as the CGFNS, is a not-for-profit organization that completes credential evaluations for professional nurses, authenticates and verifies nurse's credentials, and then issues a certification to the state board of nursing for which the nurse is applying to take their NCLEX testing with.

The CGFNS is dedicated to the registration and licensure of all overseas nurses, whether they are from English speaking countries or not. In order for nurses to obtain their credentials they must take the NCLEX (National Council of Licensing's Exam) and pass an English language test.

At the writing of this book (July 2016), the credentialing service had a fee of $350. There is also an additional English proficiency report that has an $85 fee. This report is required by 14% of the states in the

United States. There is also a fee for re-evaluation, additional reports, additional report recipients, and expedited service.

For the evaluation you will need to provide your license information, registration information, and diploma information. You must also have a comprehensive educational transcript. All professional schools must be included in this report.

The English language tests that you may take include the TOEFL (Test of English as a Foreign Language) or the IELTS (International English Language Testing System). One of these exams must be completed if your education and textbooks were not printed or spoken in the English Language.

After you have passed the NCLEX and one of the English language tests the CGFNS will review your Visa Application, and if acceptable, will issue you a Work Visa Screen. To obtain this screen you must also visit the consular officer and inform him/her of your intentions to work in the United States.

To do all of this you must also have a Visa Sponsor, which is a travel company that will assist you in obtaining all the requirements for your Work Visa. Usually this will be attached to you during the time that you work for that travel company. (CFGNS, 2016)

Work VisaScreen®

The VisaScreen® is an official document that you will receive from the CGFNS that states that you meet all the legal requirements to work inside the United States and that you are an RN (Registered Nurse). This means that your educational credentials and your competency testing meet the standards for all nurses who wish to obtain a job. The VisaScreen® also certifies that you have met the standards set by the Department of Homeland Security.

This screen will certify that you have taken and passed a language test such as the TOEFL or the IELTS, as described in the section above.

For the VisaScreen® you will need to have a license for registered nursing that is not restricted, transcripts from your nursing program showing that you have passed the national council of nursing's licensing exam, and obtained a sponsor.

It is also important to note that if you wish to become a resident of some states, you have a legal and clear nursing license you may be able to obtain a CGFNS certificate in lieu of the VisaScreen®. Related to the nursing shortage, the Department of Homeland security is making it easier for nurses who have a nursing license in another country to get a United States license and this has shortened some of the processes necessary for immigration.

One thing to remember in this process is that there are only limited amounts of Work VisaScreen® processed every year. The selection is based on the country in which you were born; therefore, going to nursing school in the United States under a student visa does not always guarantee you a work visa.

After all of this is completed you are on your way to getting a great job as a registered nurse in the United States. And remember that after you get a year's worth of experience you will have many opportunities to travel and work as a traveling nurse all over the United States. There is no better way to have a career and work at the same time! (VisaScreen®, 2016)

English Language Testing

When you make an application for your work visa, one of the things they will want to know if you did not go to a school with English textbooks is if you are proficient in the English language. This is accomplished by taking either the IELTS or the TOEFL test. This is a must before you can get a job as a registered nurse.

IELTS stands for "International English Language Testing System." It is a test of English language proficiency. It is jointly managed by the University of Cambridge ESOL Examinations, the British Council, and IDP Education Australia and was established in 1989. There are two versions of this test: the Academic Version (which nurses and medical professionals must pass), and a General Training Version used by more than 2,000 universities in the United States.

The IELTS incorporates a variety of accents and writing styles that are presented in text materials in order to minimize linguistic bias. The IELTS tests the ability to listen, read, write, and speak the English Language. Each candidate is scored in four modules: Listening, Reading, Writing, and Speaking. It is scored on a scale from 1 to 9 with a "9" being an expert user. All nurses must score a total of at least 7, classified as a "Good User," which means that he or she has an operational command of the language, though with occasional inaccuracies, inappropriateness, and misunderstandings in some situations, and that he or she generally handles complex language well and understands detailed reasoning. (IELTS, 2016)

The TOEFL (Test of English as a Foreign Language) evaluates the potential success of an individual to use and understand Standard American English at a college level. It is required for non-native applicants at many English-speaking colleges and universities. Additionally, institutions such as government agencies, businesses, or scholarship programs may require this test. A TOEFL score is valid for two years and then is deleted from the official database. Colleges and universities usually consider only the most recent TOEFL score.

The Internet-Based Test was introduced in late 2005 and has progressively replaced both the computer-based test and the paper-based tests. The IBT is now in use in the United States, Canada, France, Germany, and Italy.

Although the demand for test seats was very high and candidates had to wait for months, it is now possible to take the test within one to four weeks in most countries. The four-hour test consists of four sections, each measuring mainly one of the basic language skills (although some tasks may require multiple skills), focusing on language used in an academic, and higher education environment. Note taking is allowed during the IBT. The test cannot be taken more than once a week.

The reading section consists of 3–5 long passages and questions about the passages. The passages are on academic topics; they are the kind of material that might be found in an undergraduate university textbook. Students answer questions about main ideas, details, inferences, sentence restatements, sentence insertion, vocabulary, function, and overall ideas. New types of questions in the IBT require paraphrasing, filling out tables, or completing summaries. Generally, prior knowledge of the subject under discussion is not necessary to come to the correct answer, though a prior knowledge may help.

The listening section consists of six long passages and questions about the passages. The passages consist of two student conversations and four academic lectures or discussions. The questions ask the students to determine main ideas, details, function, stance, inferences, and overall organization.

The speaking section consists of six tasks, two independent tasks and four integrated tasks. In the two independent tasks students must answer opinion questions about some aspect of academic life. In two integrated reading, listening, and speaking tasks students must read a passage, listen to a passage, and speak about how the ideas in the two passages are related. In two integrated listening and speaking tasks students must listen to long passages and then summarize and offer opinions on the information in the passages. Test takers are expected to convey information, explain ideas, and defend opinions clearly, coherently, and accurately.

The writing section consists of two tasks, one integrated task and one independent task. In the integrated task students must read an academic passage, listen to an academic passage, and write about how the ideas in the two passages are related. In the independent task students must write a personal essay.

It should be noted that at least one of the sections of the test will include extra, uncounted material. Educational Testing Service includes extra material to try it out for future tests. If the test taker is given a longer section he must work hard on all of the materials because he does not know which material counts and which material is extra. For example, if there are four reading passages instead of three, three of the passages will count and one of the passages will not be counted. It is possible that the uncounted passage could be any of the four passages.

The paper-based test is given in areas where the Internet-based and computer-based tests are not available. Because test takers cannot register at the testing center on the test date, they must register in advance, using the registration form provided in the Supplemental Paper TOEFL Bulletin. They should register in advance of the given deadlines to ensure a place because the test centers have limited seating and may fill up early. Tests are administered only several times each year.

With the Internet-based test nurses must make a score of 76. The computer-based test is scored on a scale from 0 to 300. Each of the four sections is given a total of 30 points, and then these are all added together to get the total score. For the computer test you must make 207, and for the written you must make a 540.

There were many changes made in 2006, including: (1) Overall, passages have become longer; (2) Part 1 has fewer questions involving photo descriptions; (3) The Listening Section hires not only North

American English speakers but also British, Australian, and New Zealand English speakers. The ratio is 25% each for American, Canadian, British and Australian-New Zealand pronunciation; (4) Part 6 no longer contains the error spotting task, which has been criticized as unrealistic in a corporate environment but instead adopts the task wherein the test taker fills in the blanks in incomplete sentences, and (5) Part 7 contains not only single-passage questions but also double-passage questions wherein the test taker has to read and compare the two related passages such as e-mail correspondence.

Another change in 2007 added speaking and writing tests, and some changes were made to the reading and listening test as well that emphasized knowledge of grammatical rules.

This test will take you two hours to complete and consists of 200 questions. Half of the questions are on listening comprehension and the other half is on reading comprehension. Each person receives a score from 5 to 495 on each part for a total of 10 to 990. Nurses make a score of 725.

After you have completed and passed one of these tests and the NCLEX you can apply to the state board of nursing in which you reside. Through the CGFNS you will then be given your work visa. After you have received your nursing license you are on your way to one year of nursing experience, and then down the road to a travel nursing job. (TOEFL, 2016)

The NCLEX

The NCLEX is the National Council Licensure Examination, which is used to test the competency of all nurses who have completed their required educational program at an accredited university. This test is also required of all foreign-born nurses who wish to come to the United States to practice. This test will be a part of your Work Visa Screen.

This test of 265 questions is performed on a computer. Once you have reached the amount of questions determined by the national council of nursing to prove that you are competent, your test will announce that you have completed the test. Some nurses have gone to 75 and passed, and some nurses have gone to 75 and failed. Some nurses have gone to 265 and passed and some not. Wherever the test shuts off, you really never know how you have done until you get your results in the mail.

The NCLEX-RN (National Council Licensure Examination-Registered Nurse) is a computer-adaptive test (CAT) of entry-level nursing competence. Passing the exam is required of candidates for licensure as a Registered Nurse (RN) by all US state and territorial Boards of Nursing.

The NCLEX-RN and NCLEX-PN examinations are developed and owned by the National Council of State Boards of Nursing, Inc. (NCSBN). NCSBN administers these examinations on behalf of its member boards, which consist of the boards of nursing in the 50 states, the District of Columbia, and four U.S. territories: American Samoa, Guam, Northern Mariana Islands, and the Virgin Islands. This test is given only in English.

To ensure public protection, each board of nursing requires a candidate for licensure to pass the appropriate NCLEX examination: NCLEX-RN for registered nurses and the NCLEX-PN for practical/vocational nurses. NCLEX examinations are designed to test the knowledge, skills, and abilities essential to the safe and effective practice of nursing at the entry-level.

NCLEX examinations are provided in a computerized adaptive testing (CAT) format and are presently administered by Pearson VUE in their network of Pearson Professional Centers (PPC). Authorized testing centers are located throughout USA and in selected foreign countries, including the most recently approved—the Philippines and Mexico. Click on their external link and visit the NCSBN for a list of approved countries where the NCLEX exam is given.

All items are developed and validated, using the expertise of practicing nurses, educators, and regulators from throughout the country. The content of the items of the NCLEX examinations is based on a practice analysis conducted every three years. All students considering taking the NCLEX and/or CGFNS exams must keep in mind that the exams are about basic nursing intervention, and not about nursing intervention beyond the level of practice of any entry-level nurse.

The two most important elements when considering and discerning the most correct answer are whether the answer is part of an intervention that is "safe" and "effective." Students should use this as a guideline: if an answer doesn't have the elements of a "safe" and "effective" intervention, whether seeking the physical and/or psychosocial integrity of a patient, that answer cannot be the "best" answer. It can be partially correct, but most likely it is not the best answer of the multiple possible answers. (NCLEX, 2016)

After you have taken a nursing competency test, English language competency test, obtained a sponsor and have applied for your work visa screen you are well on your way to becoming a travel nursing RN. Once you have that license in hand and work at your sponsored hospital for up to a year you will have the chance to take your skills on the road fulltime with a travel nursing job. Travel nursing RN jobs are not only financially rewarding, but they offer the best way to get around and visit the different parts of the United States.

~*~

Travel Companies Who Assist Foreign Nurses

Adex Medical Staffing – Specializes in providing quality health care and medical staffing services travel and per diem projects. www.adexmedicalstaffing.com/internationalnurses/

Assignment America – They can help you achieve your personal and professional goals in an exciting U.S. nursing career. As part of the Cross Country Healthcare family of companies, Assignment America draws on more than 40 years of experience working with the top health care facilities in the United States. www.assignmentamerica.com

Cirrus Medical Staffing – At Cirrus Medical Staffing, they specialize in the placement of traveling medical professionals. If you're ready to earn top dollar, leverage your skills, and enjoy the adventure of a lifetime, this is where your journey begins. www.cirrusmedicalstaffing.com

Global Healthcare Group – Travel nursing agency with branches and affiliates in the UK, Canada, Philippines, India, South Africa, and the Middle East. www.globalhealthcaregroup.com

Medliant – In the business of supplying international nurses to staffing companies all over the United States. www.medliant.com

O'Grady Peyton – Learn more about the allied health and nurse employment opportunities at O'Grady Peyton. We offer travel nursing jobs to North American nurses and long-term positions for health care professionals from many other countries. www.ogradypeyton.com

Parallon Workforce Solutions – High paying per diem shifts, travel assignments, and full-time positions for Registered Nurses and Healthcare Professionals are available now! Parallon Workforce Solutions offers you the best opportunities, benefits and rates in the industry! www.parallonjobs.com

Premier Healthcare Professionals – When you work in the U.S. with PHP, they will assist you with the hassles of relocation so you can focus on enjoying life and practicing your profession. Their dedicated staff will arrange your placement, relocation, housing, insurance, and provide continued support throughout your assignment. www.travelphp.com

Strategic Healthcare – Strategic offers you a variety of unique opportunities to live and work in new places while expanding your professional horizons. Their experienced licensing, immigration, and housing specialists coordinate your pre-employment arrangements and advise you on all aspects of your relocation to the United States. www.strategic-healthcare.com/international-programs.html

Worldwide Travel Nursing – WTS has many travel nursing jobs around the world and is the only travel nursing company that provides true travel nursing jobs to the travel nursing industry worldwide! www.worldwidetravelstaffing.com

*** References ***

CFGNS. (2016). Facts retrieved from CFGNS: http://www.cgfns.org/services/ces-professional-report/

IELTS. (2016, July 22. Facts retrieved from Wikipedia, a public domain governed by a General Public License: http://en.wikipedia.org/wiki/IELTS

NCLEX. (2016, July 22). Facts retrieved from Wikipedia, a public domain governed by a General Public License: http://en.wikipedia.org/wiki/NCLEX

TOEFL. (2016, July 22). Facts retrieved from Wikipedia, a public domain governed by a General Public License: http://en.wikipedia.org/wiki/TOEFL

VisaScreen®. (2016). Facts retrieved from CGFNS: http://www.cgfns.org/services/visascreen/

Chapter Fifteen

Traveling To A Foreign Country

Go to foreign countries and you will get to know the good things one possesses at home. (Johann Wolf)

The travel thirst of many nurses might be quenched by thirteen week contracts at hospitals all over the United States. For some however, even more adventure is required. This chapter is for them. We will discuss options for nurses who wish to work outside the US as well as practice possibilities outside of the traditional hospital environment. This chapter is broken down into several sections: (1) Opportunities to work within the healthcare systems of other countries, (2) Opportunities to work for the United States government in other countries, (3) Opportunities in International relief and development, and (4) Opportunities in international transport and industrial nursing.

Nurses considering employment abroad need to be aware of the realities of international nursing practice before committing the substantial time and financial resources required to make this possibility a reality. Working conditions, scope of practice, and salary vary widely around the world. In many locations, nurses need to be able to suture or do minor surgical procedures while in still others, skills common to US nurses like peripheral IV placement might be done solely by physicians. In general, the wide variety of allied health professions that exist in the US may be very limited or nonexistent in other countries. The work done by physical, occupational, and respiratory therapists is commonly split between physicians and nurses. Nurses may be expected to run ventilators, draw Arterial Blood Gases, and perform other skills that are done in the US by other professional groups.

Before considering an overseas assignment, a nurse should ask themselves several questions to ensure they and their loved ones are prepared for them to work abroad.

Question #1: Why do I want to go overseas? Answer this before reading further! Good answers include: To see the world, to explore a different practice environment, to find adventure and romance! Bad answers to that question include: running from the law, running from the tax man, or running from the ex!

Question #2: Am I comfortable with a change in my social and family life? Are you okay with being away from family and friends for a year or more? Sure, you'll make new friends, and with instant communication just a SIM card away this challenge is easier than it used to be, but the distance remains. You might be joining your Aunt Berthas 90th birthday party or your sister's wedding via Facetime while the rest of the family is there in person.

Question #3: Do I have the financial resources to do this? Salaries for nurses in much of the world are significantly lower than in the United States. Those working in relief and development may get only a stipend or expenses covered. What will you do about mortgage or student loan payments? If you're saving for retirement, will you be able to continue your contributions to your IRA while working abroad? Taxes are another concern. The IRS requires every American citizen to file a tax return, regardless of where they are residing. Enforcement of this law has been stepped up in recent years. While there may be some tax benefits to residing outside of the United States for an extended period of time, you will need to consult a tax professional regarding taxes both for the United States and for the country you are working in.

Question #4: What will I come back to? Reentry into your home society and family group may be difficult. Friends have gotten married, divorced, elected, or paroled. You've had adventures that they may not seem interested in. Your travel nurse recruiter might question whether you're still current in your specialty and you might very well decide that where and who you left, is not where and who you wish to return to.

While your family and friends might think your desire to work overseas is a bit off, there is a network of nurses who are doing or have done the same thing. Seek them out at work, on social media, and at conferences. Get tips and referrals from people who have done this before.

Opportunities Within National Health Systems

It might help to research the structure of the healthcare system in the countries you would consider working in. An in-depth discussion of national health care programs is well outside the scope of this book, but generally speaking, the United States is almost unique among developed nations in not having a national healthcare system. Most nations have a system of government hospitals and clinics that are supplemented with private facilities. While all of these might use foreign nurses, as a general rule the salaries in government facilities will be lower than that found in the private sector. It is important to discuss with a nursing agency recruiter whether you want to work within the private or public systems of a given country

Before any further discussion, we must clarify two different but related issues: Licensure and Immigration.

Licensure is permission to practice. Similar to a nursing license issued by a State Board of Nursing, every country has an agency that regulates the practice of nursing. This is the agency that will review your educational transcripts and other documents to determine if you meet the minimum requirements to practice as a nurse in that country.

The immigration agency is the entity that may grant permission to remain in and work in the country. This agency will also review your documents and those of your potential employer to determine if you qualify for a work visa. Every country does this differently and sets their own requirements for issuing a visa. Traveling nurses may be eligible for a wide variety of visa categories depending on education, experience, age, and even nursing specialty. Immigration eligibility might even be obtained based on your ancestry.

In order to practice nursing in another country, you must satisfy the requirements of BOTH licensure and immigration. For most countries, licensure is addressed first, and once that is obtained, then immigration. Reputable nurse staffing agencies in most countries will have staff to guide prospective employees through these processes.

The Middle East, particularly Saudi Arabia, was once known as a high paying destination for American RNs, with Helen Ziegler and associates sending thousands there in the 80's. Increasing pay rates in the US as well as the changing geopolitical landscape have decreased this perception somewhat.

The region remains a popular destination however, with the United

Arab Emirates, including Dubai, Abu Dhabi and Qatar as the more popular destinations. Cleveland Clinic opened an Abu Dhabi facility in 2015 and, along with Sidra Health System in Qatar, continues to recruit significant numbers of overseas nurses. In Saudi Arabia, the hospitals are run by the government or by the military. Western staff in Saudi Arabia or Kuwait typically live in fenced compounds with other westerners. When outside these compounds, there are restrictions on attire and movement. Female nurses, or any females for that matter, may not drive in Saudi Arabia. Foreigners in the UAE don't typically face as many restrictions. Alcohol is widely available and western women are exempted from Islamic dress requirements. Travelers in the UAE would be well served though to remember they are working in a conservative area. In 2010, a British couple were imprisoned for one month in Dubai after being convicted of kissing in public. While many agencies can send you to the Middle East, Helen Ziegler is still the consensus expert for placements in the region. The complex licensure and immigration processes found in practically all the Middle East countries are best undertaken with the help of an agency recruiter.

Outside of the Middle East, the most common destinations for American nurses tend to be the English speaking "western" countries. These include Australia, New Zealand, and the UK. These countries typically require a Bachelor's degree in Nursing. Some countries, particularly the UK, require that the educational program be a certain number of lecture and clinical hours in length. This degree must be the "Pre-licensure educational preparation." In other words, the degree you obtained to get your nursing license. This means that Associates degree prepared RNs who then return to school to obtain a Bachelor's are not eligible for licensure in most countries. Nurses who obtained their degree through distance education programs are also typically not eligible for licensure. Associates degree prepared RNs might be able to work in these countries through opportunities found later in this chapter. Below is a list of the most common English speaking destinations for American nurses, the education required for licensure, and the web addresses of both licensure and immigration agencies. The requirements for working and living in these countries change rapidly. Most will have nurse staffing agencies similar to those found in the US to help you through the process. Aside from the Working Holiday Visa discussed later, most of these countries are seeking nurses on a "permanent" basis rather than the 13 week travel contract so common in the United States.

Australia, Canada, New Zealand, Bermuda, and Ireland require that you have a BSN; the UK will take either a 3-year Diploma Nurse or a BSN. The licensing agency for Australia can be found at www.nursingmidwiferyboard.gov.au and immigration can be found at www.border.gov.au. The licensing agency for Canada can be found at www.nnas.ca, and immigration information can be found at www.cic.gc.ca. The New Zealand council for nursing can be found at www.immigration.govt.nz. The Bermuda nursing council can be found at www.bnc.bm and the immigration department can be found at www.gov.bm/department/immigration. The UK board can be found at www.nmc.org.ul with the immigration depart at www.gove.uk

Younger nurses might be eligible for what is known as a Working Holiday Visa. Offered by several countries, this visa allows Americans up to age 30 (35 for New Zealand) to remain in the country and work for one year. This is a very simple and inexpensive visa to obtain. Several agencies will process these visas; among the most experienced is the British University North America Club (www.bunac.org). Young nurses who wish to use this service should do so sooner rather than later, as Working Holiday programs are subject to change or elimination based on the prevailing political winds.

Opportunities to Work for the US government Abroad

Perhaps you want to combine working as a nurse abroad with serving your country. Nurses with a Bachelor's degree might consider joining the military. Nurses in the Armed Forces are commissioned officers who enjoy a great deal of respect and a dynamic working environment with plenty of opportunity for professional advancement. For nurses who want to travel while maintaining a full time job at home, the National Guard and Reserve might be an ideal solution. While the military offers many opportunities, it is not for everyone. Many do not like the structured lifestyle the military requires or find that the salary is quite low compared to the civilian world.

Many nurses may not be aware that The US Public Health Service is also a Uniformed Service. While most of the USPHS Commissioned Corps nurses work at facilities throughout the United States, there are sometimes opportunities to work overseas. Such an event took place recently when the Centers for Disease Control, a part of the USPHS responded to the 2014-2015 outbreak of Ebola Virus Disease in West Africa.

Nurses who don't want to make the years long commitment required for military service might consider work as a Department of Defense Civilian Employee. The DOD employs almost 800,000 civilians around the world in various capacities. DOD civilian nurses work alongside military staff or other federal employees to provide care in various settings. The largest concentrations of DOD civilian nurses overseas are found in Germany at Landstuhl Regional Medical Center. LRMC is the primary medical facility for US Military members and their families across Europe, Africa, and the Middle East. It was among the first facilities outside the United States certified as a Trauma Center by The American College of Surgeons. Openings for civilian RNs can often be found at smaller DOD facilities throughout Europe and also in Asia as well. Civilian RNs are often employed on a 1–2 year contract basis, including an allowance for relocation and housing. DOD civilian positions are often open to Associates Degree prepared RNs. The DOD also has frequent openings for Licensed Practical Nurses, presenting that group with a rare international travel opportunity. DOD civilian positions can be found at www.usajobs.gov. Be aware that the recruiting process for these positions can be quite long. Some nurses report a full year passing between when they send in their application and when an offer is received.

The US Department of State also has periodic openings for nurses in international locations. These are also found at www.usajobs.gov. The staff nurses typically employed in US Embassies abroad are most often recruited locally, but MSN or DNP prepared Nurse Practitioners may apply to the Foreign Service Medical Provider Program for worldwide placements.

Opportunities in International Relief and Development

Perhaps you saw a video of a flood or earthquake on your friend's Facebook feed. Maybe you want to get back some of the feeling of helping others that motivated you to go to nursing school in the first place. Nurses pursue humanitarian work for a variety of reasons. Humanitarian work can be an especially rewarding field despite the lack of financial reward. It should be noted that while this chapter discusses international relief and development, we are not talking about short term volunteer postings or "mission trips." This chapter is about full time or rotational employment in the sector. Earlier in this chapter we discussed evaluating your reasons for wanting to work overseas. Nurses considering working in the humanitarian sector should spend extra time discerning their motivation as well as their resources and the impact on family and friends back home. This is important as unlike most of the opportunities presented in this chapter, you may very well find yourself working in an area with very limited or no infrastructure, with colleagues who may not speak your language and whom you are trusting with your safety.

While often lumped together under the category of humanitarian aid work, relief and development are in fact two distinct disciplines. Relief is typically short-term efforts in response to an acute event. A flood, a war, an outbreak, etc. with staff moving from one crisis to the next. The effort is time limited and focused on emergent care. This is field hospitals and helicopters. Development on the other hand is typically longer-term focused and may include Health System development or strengthening, public health education campaigns, or even research. This is vaccinating children and building latrines. Relief is the sexy headline grabbing work. Development is the work that will improve more lives in the long run. There is overlap, as many crises today seem open ended in nature. Agencies that formerly did only relief work now have development projects and vice versa. Work in the humanitarian sector is typically done by government entities like the US Agency for International Development (USAID), Intergovernmental groups like the United Nations, and by Non-Governmental Organizations (NGOs) such as The Red Cross and Doctors Without Borders. There are literally thousands of NGOs that work in the humanitarian arena. Job postings for this sector are found on the website for the UN Office for the Coordination of Humanitarian Affairs at www.reliefweb.int. Training opportunities can be found on the same website. Nurses who wish to work in this area should consider taking courses in tropical medicine and public health, logistics and International Humanitarian Law. Short courses on these topics are readily available throughout the US and abroad. The prestigious London School of Hygiene & Tropical Medicine (www.lshtm.ac.uk) offers a Diploma in Tropical Nursing.

There have been many volumes written on the ethics and efficacy of humanitarian work. While that discussion is outside the scope of this book, at a minimum, you should carefully investigate any potential employer before agreeing to work for them. Questions that might be asked about a prospective employer include: (1) Does the organization have a political or religious mission? Many NGOs are religious in nature. (2) If so, is it a mission I can work with? If you're an atheist, an evangelical Christian group might not be the best fit. (3) What countries do they work in? How long have they worked there? Long established projects and organizations might be better for a nurse new to the field. (4) How are they funded? Are their projects sustainable? Choose an organization that isn't at risk of running out of funds during the course of your employment. Check charitynavigator.org or similar websites to evaluate how they spend the donated dollar.

What is the plan if something goes wrong? Work in this sector is not without an element of personal risk. This is demonstrated by the infection of clinicians responding to the recent Ebola Virus Disease outbreak in West Africa, as well as by the recent targeting of medical facilities by hostile factions in the Syrian civil war. With proper planning and preparedness, these risks can be minimized. Reputable agencies working in high crime or conflict prone areas should contract with security and evacuation companies like Global Rescue Inc. (www.globalrescue.com). Reasonable personal safety precautions should also be taken by the nurse working in low resource settings. Pre-employment vaccinations, anti-malarial regimen adherence, and attention to basic hygiene matters will make your tenure safer.

Opportunities for nurses in International Transport and Industrial Settings

There has been an increase in the need for medical care in industrial settings. Many mining entities, oil and gas companies, and other extractive industries have large amounts of employees working onsite in many foreign countries. The countries these companies are based in often require a minimum set of medical skills and equipment be available onsite. In the past, many of these positions were filled by paramedics and as such may appeal to RNs with an EMS background. Recently, an increase in postings requiring a Registered Nurse has been seen. Like humanitarian work, industrial settings are not for everyone. A nurse might find themselves in a mining camp in The Congo, or the only caregiver for 150 people on an oilrig in the middle of the ocean for five weeks. If that sounds good to you, consider taking a Helicopter Underwater Escape Training (HUET) course. Such training is required for almost all industrial positions. Medical professionals are not typically employed by the drilling or mining company themselves, but rather by specialist agencies like Remote Medical International (www.remotemedical.com) or International SOS (www.internationalSOS.com), in an arrangement familiar to most American traveling nurses employed by staffing agencies rather than hospitals. An oilrig not extreme enough for your nursing career? How about the South Pole? There are rare openings for nurses to work in Antarctica through the US Antarctic Program medical contractor the University of Texas Medical Branch. These postings are highly competitive and can be found at www.utmb.edu/polar.

International transport nursing is a small but growing field. Flight nursing is a way to see much of the world and interact with other healthcare systems without actually living abroad. International air ambulance companies transport patients who were traveling in foreign lands and became ill or injured. They also transport patients seeking specialty care in the United States or abroad. This is typically done in specially modified fixed wing aircraft that are configured to function as an airborne ICU. Flight teams usually consist of a Registered Nurse and a Paramedic or Respiratory Therapist. Nurses considering working in long range fixed wing flight environments must consider several things. How comfortable are they with clinical autonomy using Medical Director approved protocols? Can they work well in small groups in tight spaces for extended periods? While fixed wing flight nursing does not have the weight limits required for helicopter work, a certain level of physical fitness is required for the job due to heavy lifting and confined spaces. The minimum qualifications are five years of ICU or ER experience. Having both ICU and ER experience will make a candidate much more attractive to Air Ambulance companies. Postings and further information about flight nursing can be found at the website of the Air and Surface Transport Nurses Association (www.astna.org) as well as at www.flightweb.com.

Cruise ship work really floats the boat of many nurses. While the allure of tropical islands and other exotic ports of call is tempting, there is a lot of work to be done on cruise ships. Most cruise ships afloat today have 3–5 nurses and 2–3 physicians for a population of up to 6,000 passengers and crew. Nurses should have 3–5 years of critical care or ER experience. A typical day starts with early morning clinics for both passengers and crew. Then there will be office hours, water supply testing, and crew physicals. Once all that work is done, there might be a couple of hours for the nurses who aren't on call to go to the beach or to Barcelona or to Glacier Bay. Nurses who work on cruise ships must be as comfortable in a customer service environment as they are with critical care procedures. This becomes especially challenging when confronting a norovirus outbreak that is causing vomiting and diarrhea among hundreds of guests. Nurses on ship are Deck Officers who have extensive privileges, including a private stateroom and the services of a room steward. You have almost no expenses while onboard and can thus save more of your salary than at a land based contract. Most cruise lines employ nurses on a 4 month on/2 month off or similar contract. Holland America, a unit of the Carnival conglomerate, occasionally has openings for part time nurses. Postings for these openings can be found at the websites of various cruise lines.

The industrial and transport sector isn't all norovirus and oilrigs. Many of the larger resort hotel chains like Club Med (www.clubmed.us) employ nurses on a seasonal basis to care for staff and guests. If you like your nursing career with lots of ups and downs, amusement parks like roller coaster paradise Cedar Point and family destination Disneyworld hire nurses to work alongside medics in the parks. Check the website of your favorite park in late winter for details of summer season hiring.

For those who seek the adventure of an international assignment yet still desire the comfort of remaining within sight of the Red, White, and Blue, there are quasi-international opportunities out there for intrepid nurses. The US Virgin Islands and Guam have a high demand for nurses due to a chronic shortage of local staff. Each provides lush tropical beaches without the need for a passport or immigration paperwork. Guam Memorial Hospital Authority recruits through their website at www.gmha.org. The US Virgin Islands can be reached through many travel nursing agencies.

If all this information seems overwhelming, that's understandable. There is literally a world of opportunity out there for the adventurous nurse. You've already completed the hardest part of getting a job overseas by graduating from nursing school. Asking yourself the questions at the beginning of this chapter should give you a sense of where you want to go and why. Then determine what setting you wish to work in, and go for it. Remember to pack your stethoscope!

~*~

This chapter was authored by Aaron Highfill, RN, CFRN. Growing up in a military family, Aaron comes by his wanderlust naturally. He started in healthcare as an EMT-Basic in 1996, and has worked his way up through LPN to finally obtaining his RN degree. While working in the ER and Urgent Care in the cold and rainy weather, he got a call from a recruiter wanting to know if he would like to go to the Virgin Isalands. Since then, his nursing career has taken him to approximately twenty-four foreign countries, six continents, two cruise ships, one civil war and a viral pandemic as a Flight Nurse.

Chapter Sixteen

Independent Contracting

True independence and freedom can only exist in doing what's right. (Brigham Young)

Many nurses now have put on the hat of nurse entrepreneur. Getting contracts by yourself and doing your own independent contracting is a little tougher than just having an agency helping you with taxes, government dues, insurance, and getting assignments, but there are definite advantages, with more money coming into your pocket and having control over your destination.

One of the basic differences of being an independent contractor instead of an employee is that you will be receiving the IRS Form 1099 instead of a W2 form. This IRS Form 1099 shows the amount that was paid for services rendered. This form will have on it the account number (or unique number), the payer assigned to distinguish your account, the amount subject to self-employment taxes, other income, backup withholdings, and any state of local income tax withheld from the payments.

Another difference is that you will be responsible for obtaining your own contracts. Most commonly, this is done in two ways: first, by calling the hospital and seeing the availability of contracts, which they usually use for contracts, and if they would consider an independent contract, or you can contact a company that specializes in independent contracts. These companies will charge you a few dollars per hour for helping you in obtaining a "subcontract" through them. There used to be four or five companies that you could subcontract for, but in 2016, the only company that I know of is Moore Nurses (moorenurses.com).

I know, you're anxious to get down the road by yourself, but there are just a few more basics that you have to understand, such as the type of business you are going to have, formulating a business plan, creating a marketing plan, must haves for the office, and what to put into the contract. You just never know, after starting your own independent contractor business you may want to expand and let other nurses share in your happiness and wealth.

What Type of Business?

First, you need to decide what type of business you will start. There are several types, including a sole proprietor (the most common), a C-Corporation, an S-Corporation, or a limited liability corporation (LLC).

A sole proprietorship is a corporation that officially has no separate existence from its owner. Hence, the limitations of liability enjoyed by a corporation do not apply. All debts of the business are debts of the owner. It is a "sole" proprietor in the sense that the owner has no partners. A sole proprietorship essentially means that a person does business in their own name and there is only one owner. A sole proprietorship is not a corporation; it does not pay corporate taxes, but rather the person who organized the business pays personal income taxes on the profits made, making accounting much simpler. A sole proprietorship need not worry about double taxation like a corporation would have to.

A business structured as a sole proprietorship will likely have a hard time creating capital, since shares of the business cannot be sold, and there is a smaller sense of legitimacy relative to a business that is organized as a corporation or limited liability company. Hiring employees may also be difficult. This form of business will have unlimited liability; therefore, if the business is sued, it is the proprietor's problem.

Another disadvantage of a sole proprietorship is that as a business becomes successful, the risks accompanying the business tend to grow. To minimize those risks, a sole proprietor has the option of forming a limited liability company. Most sole proprietors will register a trade name or "Doing Business As." This allows the proprietor to do business with a name other than their legal name, and it also allows them to open a business account with banking institutions.

A C-corporation is a form of corporation that meets the IRS requirements to be taxed under Subchapter C-of the Internal Revenue Code. Most major companies are incorporated under a C-corporation.

After the corporation is created, it becomes its own entity and has an indefinite lifespan, as long as the yearly filing fee is paid. This is what you would want to file if you were starting a staffing agency that would have several employees.

The main difference between S and C is the fact that a C-corporation is taxed a Federal Corporate Income tax, whereas an S-corporation is not. It may also have an unlimited amount of shareholders, as well as foreign shareholders, unlike S-corporations.

In order to accomplish the task of becoming a C-Corp, you will need to choose an available business name that complies with your state's corporation rules, appoint the initial directors of your corporation, file formal paperwork, usually called "articles of incorporation," and pay a filing fee that ranges from $100 to $800, depending on the state in which you incorporate, create corporate "bylaws," which lay out the operating rules for your corporation, hold the first meeting of the board of directors, issue stock certificates to the initial shareholders of the corporation, and obtain licenses and permits that may be required for your business.

An S-Corporation is taxed as a joint venture, while at the same time it enjoys the benefit of incorporation. This means that, while the S-Corporation itself pays no federal income tax, the shareholders of the S-Corporation pay federal income tax on their proportionate share of the S-Corporation's income. In other words, any profits earned by the corporation will not be taxed at the corporate level, but instead will be taxed only at the level of the individual shareholders.

Unlike C-Corp dividends, which are taxed at the federal rate of 15.00%, S-Corp dividends are taxed at the shareholder's marginal tax rate. However, the C-Corp dividend is subject to "double-taxation." The income is first taxed at the corporate level before it is distributed as a dividend. The dividend is then taxed at the personal capital gains rate when issued to the shareholder.

S-Corp Distributions are only taxed once at the marginal rate of each shareholder who received a distribution. Additionally, the S-Corp shareholder will pay taxes on the S-Corp earnings, whether or not a distribution is made. Having S-Corporation status can prove a huge benefit for a corporation. The corporation can pass income directly to shareholders and avoid the double taxation that is inherent with the dividends of public companies, while still enjoying the advantages of the corporate structure.

In order to qualify, a corporation must be a small business corporation. Requirements that must be met include the fact that it must be a domestic corporation, must have no more than 100 shareholders, and all of the shareholders must be citizens of the United States. The corporation also must have only one class of stock, and profits and losses must be allocated to shareholders proportionately to each one's interest in the business.

If a corporation meets the foregoing requirements, its shareholders may file Form 2553 with the IRS. The Form 2553 must be signed by all of the corporation's shareholders. If a corporation that has elected to be treated as an S-Corporation ceases to meet the requirements, the corporation will lose its S-Corporation status.

A Limited Liability Corporation is a legal form of business offering limited liability to its owners. It is similar to a corporation and is often a more flexible form of ownership, especially suitable for smaller companies with restricted numbers of owners.

An LLC allocates for the flexibility of a sole proprietorship or partnership arrangement within the structure of limited liability, such as that approved for corporations. A benefit of an LLC over a limited partnership is that the rules and regulations required for forming and registering LLCs are much easier than the requirements most states place on developing and managing corporations. Most LLCs will, however, decide to implement an Operating Agreement or Limited Liability Company Agreement to provide for the authority of the company, and such arrangements are normally more multifaceted than a corporation's statutes.

One reason an industry might prefer to be planned out as an LLC is to circumvent dual assessment of taxes. A conventional corporation is taxed on its income, and then when the profits are dispersed to the owners of the corporation or shareholders, those dividends are also taxed. With an LLC, income of the LLC is not taxed, but each owner of the LLC is taxed, based on its pro rata allocable portion of the LLC's taxable income, apart from whether any distributions to the associates are made. This single level of taxation can lead to significant savings over the corporate form.

Another underlying motive that a company might choose to be arranged as an LLC is to take advantage of the tax classification flexibility that LLCs allow. A new business facing losses might opt to function as a sole proprietorship or partnership in order to bypass those losses to the owners. A slightly more established business might operate as an S-corporation to save on self-employment taxes. A large, mature business with many owners might operate as a C corporation.

Formulating A Business Plan

Your business plan will need to include an executive summary, general company description, products and services, an operation plan, management and organization, a personal financial statement, startup expenses and capitalization, a financial plan, and refining the plan.

The executive summary actually needs to be written last. It should include everything that you would put into a five-minute interview, including the fundamentals of the proposed business, what your services will be, who your customers will be, who the owners are, and what you think the future holds for your business. This summary needs to be KISSed…Keep It So Simple!

The general company description needs to include the fact that you are a registered nurse, providing services to hospitals, and how you will provide those services. You will need a mission statement, usually 40 words or less, which explains your reason for starting this company and what philosophies have guided you to make the decision to strike out on your own.

Next, you will need to state your goals and objectives. What goal do you have for your company? Do you want to be in the Fortune 500, or do you just want to provide great service to others, giving them quality service instead of quantity? This will depend on whether or not you decide to remain a sole proprietor or if you incorporate as a C, S, or Limited Liability Corporation.

To whom are you going to market your products? Hospitals, nursing homes, physicians' offices, surgical centers? What is the future of your company? What changes do you see in the future? How will you deal with those changes?

Also, in the goals and objectives you will need to describe why you think that your company is the best company for the job? Customer service? Experience? Skills?

This is where you will also want to state what type of corporation you have filed as and why you decided to file as that type of corporation.

Next, you will describe in-depth your products or services with technical specifications: what set of skills are available, what can you do for the hospital or medical facility? Which of these features will give you the competitive edge and exclusivity? What is the bill rate for your services? Why is your bill rate a good bargain? Hospitals are looking for the best rates and the best quality together. Can you supply that demand? (This will be discussed further in the marketing plan section).

Next is the operation plan. This will explain the day-to-day operation of the business, its home-base location, people, and processes. Some of the things you will want to include in this section are the services you will provide, quality control aspects, and customer service. Where will your home base be located? Unless you are planning on hiring a lot of nurses in a staffing company type of setting, this will be the physical location of your permanent residence. What type of licensing and insurance will you be carrying on yourself and/or personnel?

If you plan on hiring other nurses, you will need to list how many nurses you will start out with, the units of the hospital that you would like to provide services for, how to pay for their services, training methods, requirements for nurses, job description, and any need for subcontracted workers.

How will you manage your accounts receivable? You will have to formulate a plan to bill the hospital, as well as how to receive the payments. Independent contractors typically bill the hospital weekly, but payment is usually made only once a month.

Next, you should state your management members and any consults regularly used. Consults that you are smart to have available include an attorney, accountant, insurance agent, banker, nursing profession consultants, small business consultants, and mentors you feel are needed to help you run a successful business.

After that, you should explain what you believe your startup expenses are, your financial ability to assist with those expenses, and any other capital funds you have acquired or have a plan to acquire. Do your research on exactly how much it is going to cost you to start up a home office. Do you have a computer, fax machine, copy machine, and phone? A fairly inexpensive printer can do faxing, copying, and scanning. Other services can be provided through an office supply store. Once you estimate your start up expenses, it's a general rule to plan on a twenty percent financial pad for unexpected incidentals. How much do you plan to make in a year? How much do you plan to make in five years? What are your long-term financial goals? Do you plan on starting as a sole proprietor and then further incorporate into a Limited Liability Corporation or C-Corp?

Refine your plan to include the key competitive factors in the industry, capacity limits, purchasing and inventory management of supplies, and new services under development. How will you manage rapidly changing prices or costs, and how will you remain on the cutting edge with your services?

The preceding questions can be answered by taking your time and doing an in-depth look into what you really want to accomplish with your services as an independent contractor. Having this documentation will give your company more validity.

Creating a Marketing Plan

The purpose of a marketing plan is to put onto paper why you think your product is better than other products, why hospitals should hire you, why hospitals should hire your staff, and the future plans of your company. This plan will assist you in knowing where you have been and where you are going. It will keep your eyes focused on the job at hand—building your travel nursing company into a prosperous and successful business.

We are going to build this nursing company just like we take care of our patients—through assessment, planning, implementation, and evaluation. To accomplish this, first we need to assess what types of services we are going to provide, to whom we are providing those services, who are our competitors, and how the market fluctuates.

What types of services are you going to provide? This will be directly linked to what your nursing specialty is. Are you going to employ others? If you have multiple specialties, then the greatest demand will determine what services you will have the most success in providing to your clients. You will need to do some research into what hospitals you are going to target at first and determine what their needs are.

You need to research what other nursing contractors are out there and what their targeted hospitals are. What do they provide to the hospital that you could provide better? You must declare what the market is lacking in order to determine how you can fill that place.

By doing some research, you can also find out what your competitors are paying. If you explain that you are a nurse wanting to do a travel assignment and wanting to know what types of jobs they have and what the pay rates are, then you can figure a ballpark range of what the bill rate is by taking what they are paying the travel nurses and adding 20% (take the pay rate and multiply it by 1.2). You can also go to salary.com and see what the nursing salary is for that position. To get an idea of a bill rate from this you must understand that travel nurses make approximately 20% more an hour than staff nurses and the company will also get 20%. By taking the pay rate and multiplying it by 1.4 you can figure out an approximate bill rate.

Your plan will include aligning the price with the apparent value with the customer. If your price seems a little high, drop it a few dollars per hour. If you are unable to get contracts after discussing the bill rate with human resources, you may have to look at changing the price. Keep in mind also that if you provide outstanding service to a customer, you can raise your price a little on the next contract.

Snoop around and see what other competitors are out there. Are there several independent nursing companies available? Are they all providing service to one hospital, or do they cater to a group of hospitals? What are their strengths? What are their weaknesses? How can you capitalize on those weaknesses? Maybe the hospital needs a more flexible nurse…maybe they need someone to work night or weekends. Find out the need and what needs are not being provided for by other nurses and you will get your foot in the door.

You need to plan how you are going to get the word out to these hospitals. There are several ways to get the information into hospitals by using phone calls followed up with brochures and postcards telling hospitals of your new services. Carry business cards with you at all times. You never know when you are talking with people out in the community and you can tell about some hospital, clinic, or nursing home that is, "terribly short-staffed, I just don't know how they make it." Your eyes and ears should be open at all times for marketing possibilities.

What are the goals of your marketing efforts, and in what time frame do you want to accomplish them? Some nurses just want a contract for the next month, some want a contract for the next week, and some want a contract for the next year. Do you plan on helping other nurses find contracts? You might have a goal of 10 nurses this year to work in an attempt to make a good living with your company and propel it to the next level.

You also need a plan to launch your business. Follow your business plan and get your business license, get a bank account set up, and have your marketing plan ready to go. A great way to announce the beginning of your company is to place an ad in the newspaper, or better yet, send out press releases in an effort to have the media do a human interest story about why you are starting your own nursing company. If you have a self-contract, you might contact the local newspaper and offer a free article to the newspaper, with your contact and company information as a tag line.

Next, you can implement your plan in attempt to sway the client from a stage of knowledge to one of contemplation. The client needs to have confidence that you will supply their facility with the best of service.

To do this, you will need a set plan, telling when you can start, how much the bill rate will be, how you plan on doing quality control on yourself, and reinforce the fact that the independent contractors services are the best for that client. Work with the client and negotiate for the best possible deal for both you and the client.

Choose where you want to be, and beat down the doors of every hospital in that area by sending out your profile. The profile will include your resume and a skills checklist, and then start your circle to the outskirts of town. Persistence will pay off, and you will find you a job where you want if you put enough time and effort into it.

What To Put Into The Contract

Independent contracts are very similar to those of an agency nurse, but there are some differences that you need to be aware of concerning certain responsibilities: billing, insurance, and other documentation. The following is a brief description of what needs to be included.

The contractor responsibilities: A contractor (the independent contractor) is to provide nursing services in a certain area of the hospital, according to standards set forth by The Joint Commission on (TJC) and the Nursing Practice Act of the State of Idaho (my home state, you can insert yours).

The contractor certifies and will provide legal documentation of skills acquired in the past 16 years as a licensed nurse, health certificates, personal identification, company identification, and proof of liability insurance with minimum amounts of $1,000,000 per occurrence and $5,000,000 yearly.

This contract will be entered into as an independent contract with the agent not entitled to any benefits accorded to hospital employees, including workman's compensation, disability, vacation, and sick pay.

The client is responsible for providing a safe work environment, including a job description and basic orientation to medication administration, documentation, order transcription, patient safety, and on-the-job employee safety.

You may also put in there the cancellation policy for low census days, areas that you will and will not float to based on competency, any guaranteed hours, and nurse-to-patient ratios that are acceptable. Also, add in a phrase about the need to notify you two hours in advance of cancellation and you will notify them two hours in advance of unable to meet the obligation related to an illness.

Next are the financial items, including bill rates, overtime rates, weekend rates, and holiday rates. It is definitely best to keep this simple by charging a basic bill rate, overtime at 1.5 times the base pay, and holiday rates at 1.5 times the base pay. Other things that you can add, if you really feel the need to, are charge nurse pay, weekend pay, and shift differential. Just keep in mind, the more straightforward and uncomplicated the contract appears, the better it is, but don't cheat yourself either.

You should also add in a statement about when accounts are receivable. Some hospitals only pay out once a month, but by offering a 2–5% discount, some will go with a bi-weekly pay rate. Also, add a section on how much interest will be charged if the amount is not received in a timely manner. This may be anywhere from 2–5% of the total invoice for every day that is late. Also include a statement that if things go to court, lawyer fees will be asked for. You must also state when the workweek is—from Sunday to Saturday or from Monday to Sunday. You may have to be negotiable with this and go with the same schedule as the hospital has for their other employees.

Last is the termination clause. This should list how long the contract is to last and under what circumstance the contract can be terminated. The industry standard is that contracts can be cancelled with or without cause by providing thirty days written notice.

After the basic contract is written, don't be surprised if it goes through a few changes and negotiations with the hospital. It will take you an average of two weeks from the start of the negotiation process to being on the job.

Taxes and Payroll

There are several payroll taxes/costs for the independent contractor to consider ways of minimizing. I'm not including income tax in this definition. Payroll taxes usually refer to FICA, workman's comp, and unemployment insurance.

The biggest is FICA/Medicare (Federal Insurance Contributions Act), also referred to as Social Security or SSI, or in another context as the self-employment tax. Employers and employees split these taxes; employers can deduct their half as an expense. Each half is 7.65%, and together they add up to 15.3%. ICs are responsible for the entire amount, although half of it is treated as a deductible expense. There is no difference in sole proprietor and corporate treatment.

Workman's comp is technically not required for a sole proprietor (depending on the state, a corporate officer may also be exempt), but if you hire other employees, it is an absolute requirement. The hospital may require it or some other form of accident insurance. I have also read recommendations that ICs should carry workman's comp, regardless of the requirements. It costs perhaps 2% of gross payroll, so it is up to your judgment. Rules also vary quite a bit from state to state.

Unemployment insurance has a state and federal component and also accounts for about 2% of payroll. It is optional for a sole proprietor and usually a corporate officer, but not for their employees. I can't think of a good reason to pay this, and you won't be eligible for benefits anyway. It is also a cost advantage you have over an agency (you could reduce your bill rate by 2% for example to be more competitive).

The easiest way to reduce all taxes is by seeking out and taking all available legitimate expense deductions. Don't spend money just to save on taxes; that is just foolish—the more you spend the more you save theory. Deductions that a travel nurse IC should consider are meals and incidentals from Publication 1542, housing away from your tax home (leveraged with Publication 1542 schedules if you are a corporation), all travel between your tax home and the facility (if an overnight stay) at 37.5 cents a mile (or actual airfare/other costs if higher), commute miles between temporary housing and the hospital, licenses, education

R/T profession, certifications, and cell phones. Perhaps you have to hire people to maintain your home while you are away. Anything business related should be considered, including lawyer, CPA, other consultant fees, books about business, incorporation and maintenance costs, and bank fees.

Business structure directly impacts payroll taxes. S-corporations can pass some of their profits to their owners without being subject to payroll taxes. (See Business entities FAQ.) C-corps may likewise be able to figure out a scheme to do this. Be careful and get good advice, though; bonuses for officers or employees are usually considered reportable wages. Dividends to shareholders, while not subject to payroll taxes, are subject to both corporate income tax *and* personal income tax (double taxation).

In Conclusion

This is only a tip of the iceberg when it comes to the world of independent contracting. This, along with other resources including the IRS website, small business associations, and discussion boards on independent contracting or nursing entrepreneurship, will have you headed down the road to success.

***

Big thanks to Ned for allowing me to use portions of his website for some content in this chapter. Ned, RN, is the host of the Independent Contractors forum at: http://forums.delphiforums.com/ICNurse/, a forum that allows independent nurses to network, ask questions, and give advice to other independent nurses and those who wish to become independent contractors in the nursing or the broader healthcare community.

Other aspects of this chapter were written from my personal experience of being a sole proprietor of a travel nursing informational site, and being partial owner in an Internet Service Providership, which was classified as an S-Corp along with my husband's experience in both C-Corporations and Limited Liability Corporations.

Although a business plan and marketing plan are not set in stone must-haves, I do believe that it is a great way to plan out what you are trying to accomplish and have available if someone ever questions the validity of your company.

Chapter Seventeen

Traveling With Pets

Meow meow meow meow meow meow meow...
Translation – Traveling is fun especially in an RV.
(Mila & Skitzo)

For many of us our "family" also consists of a few furry children. While not impossible to travel with a pet, it is a little difficult and does cost more. For dedicated pet owners, that is a small price to pay to keep our four-legged children with us.

First of all, you need to consider what kind of pet you have. If you have a two hundred pound Saint Bernard, he is going to be much harder to travel with than if you have a two pound Chihuahua. Remember, as a traveling nurse, we try to keep things in smaller packages. The biggest problem with a larger pet also is that some apartments now have a weight limit on pets, and so do most motels. The biggest restriction that I have found is for pets that weigh over twenty pounds. They also have breed restrictions that usually restrict pit bulls, mastiffs, chows, and some boxers. Some airlines also have summer restrictions on pets with short noses such as pugs, bulldogs, and shar-pei. I also found where one airline restricts the travel of any pets during the winter months from Jackson Hole, WY; Boise, ID; and Salt Lake City, UT.

When traveling by car, you don't have as many restrictions, but it does mean a longer trip for your furry friend. There are some hotels with breed and weight restrictions, but they are usually more lenient than the airlines. The most important thing about keeping your pet in a motel room is to remember to declare your pet and pay the pet deposit. Most hotels that I have been to charge between $15 and $100 for your pet to stay the night. Sometimes they will also have a refundable pet deposit in case there is damage to the room. On the flip side, if you don't declare your pet upon arrival, then they can charge hundreds of dollars as a "fine," as if you were smoking in a non-smoking room.

A good way to find a pet-friendly hotel is through the Internet or with a downloaded phone app. Both Choice Hotels chains (Quality Inn, Comfort Inn, Clarion) have quite a few pet friendly hotels. LaQuinta has a pet-friendly app for your iPhone.

Upon arrival, always ask for the pet rules. Most hotels do not allow a pet to be in the room by themselves, especially while the housekeeping staff is in the room. These rules usually include the fact that your pet is only allowed in designated areas to do his business. Always keep your pet on a leash and keep those little green baggies handy for cleanup after Rover (a fitting name for a travel nurse' pet). Remember to dispose of the waste outside and not in the bathroom wastebaskets. It is also handy to have a towel to dry paws after being out in the grass. If you have an energetic dog, you can always ask the desk clerk if they know of a park that is close.

Along with your pet's identification on his collar, it is a good idea to get a tag with your cell phone number. Another great dog tag to have is one with his veterinarian's number included. Of course going high tech and having your pet microchipped is truly the best way to do it.

If you have to leave your pet in the room for even a short amount of time, be sure to post your cell phone number in the room, along with when you expect to be back. If your dog is a barker, this may not be a good idea, related to the fact that you may be asked to leave if Rover wakes up everyone when you go out for your midnight snack.

For traveling nurses, there are a few things that you need to check on before you embark on your next adventure. First of all, check out the state laws where you are planning your next assignment. For example, if you are wanting Hawaii in the winter, you need to realize that Hawaii has a 120-day quarantine for all pets that do not meet their "5 day or less" checklist. This 120-day quarantine also comes at a hefty price: over $1000.

Your pet should have all their shots up-to-date, and a letter of health from the veterinarian that has been taking care of your pet. To have your animal in some states parks (such as Vermont), you are required to have a letter of pet immunization before they will allow your pet inside the park. Once you get to your assignment, ask other nurses that you meet in orientation, or ask the educational supervisor, if they have a recommendation for a local veterinarian.

Although most travel companies will not let you into your apartment until just a few days before orientation, ask if you can have a few more days before to get moved in and have a few days where you are with your pet in their new environment. Of course, by having their favorite toy or cat claw station, the pet will adjust more quickly to this new place being a safe place.

One handy gadget that I found online was a KongTime automatic dispenser. It has four compartments and you can fill it with a toys or treats. This will give your pet a new toy or treat every hour or two, depending on your settings.

Before you arrive at the apartment, you should touch base with the manager of the facility or your housing coordinator about pet rent and pet deposits. Some companies cater to nurses with pets and will assist you in paying the deposit by taking it out of your check a little at a time. For pet owners that strike out on their own, they may find places that say they don't take pets will take a pet for a larger deposit. There are advantages and disadvantages to company-provided housing and traveler-provided housing. There are some companies that will encourage you to take the easy way out and leave Rover at home, but never give up! Housing can be found if you use the resources found online. With the invention of Craigslist and AirBnB, housing near your assignment is somewhat easier. Still, you may have to look at an extended-stay suite that is pet friendly. For instance, Candlewood Suites is pet friendly to pets that weigh less than 80 lbs. for a deposit of $150.

Upon arriving at the apartment, be prepared to sign a rental agreement for the stay of the pet. It will state the amount of the "pet rent" to be paid every month, along with the amount of the pet deposit. Other things that I have found on pet addendums include:

1. Pets must be kept from disturbing the peace.
2. They must be kept from damaging property.
3. Any property that is damaged will immediately be fixed or restitution will be paid to the complex/landlord.
4. The pet must be under control at all times.
5. Pets cannot be restrained by tether or chain when outside the dwelling alone.

6. Pets are not to be left at home alone for long periods of time.
7. All pet deposits made by the pet in the lawn must be taken care of promptly.
8. Food or water should always be kept indoors for the pet.
9. All pets must be vaccinated and have their records available for inspection.

Remember that you are a guest in that dwelling for a period of time. Accidents can occur, but these are best cleaned up as quickly as possible. Always keep a can of good carpet cleaner with you at all times. They have spray cans now with the scrubber at the end that make excellent spot removers. In fact, I always kept a can of it around before I got my cat. There are also other commercial "sprinkles for pets" that can be put on the carpet before vacuuming to keep pet odors down.

Part of your pet maintenance also includes protecting your pets from fleas and worms. The only flea flicker in the apartment should be on the television during football season! You definitely don't want Rover doing the butt scootin' boogie on the carpet either. These can be controlled by regular use of flea collars, sprays, and special deworming treats.

Although most of the time when we talk about traveling with animals people automatically think of dogs, more and more travelers are heading out with their feline friends. I remember one of the first times that I traveled with my rescue cat, Mila. The hotel clerk asked me what breed my dog was. I promptly answered, "Siamese." She said, "Oh, that is a cat. We don't see many people who travel with cats." They didn't even have cat treats, only doggie biscuits for a bedtime snack.

The rules are mostly the same for cats as they are for dogs, but some things are a little different, especially when starting out. It is much easier if you start out traveling when they are at a young age. We started training Mila on a leash the first time we went to the vet for her checkup. This is the second cat that I have had leash trained, but not all cats take to a leash. Be especially careful if you haven't tried leash training within the first year of life. I remember when I was a kid putting my older tomcat on a leash. Let's just say that I've never seen a cat go that ballistic.

Take them out on short rides at first, and then move to weekend trips. So far, we have made trips from Idaho to Oklahoma, from Idaho to Seattle, and from Idaho to Southern California with both of our cats, Mila and Skitzo. We have a car seat for them in which they can be harnessed in the car seat to keep them secured while traveling. Once again, this takes some time to get used to, and I would hesitate to put an older feisty cat in it.

For other cats, I would definitely suggest a cat carrier. There are hard-sided and soft-sided ones available. If you are traveling by air, it is suggested to have a soft-sided one that will fit under the seat of the airplane. The hard-sided ones are better for car trips since they can be buckled in. You don't want your furry friend to go flying in case of an accident.

Like traveling with a dog, you will want to take along spill-proof water and food bowls/dishes. Traveling with a cat also requires a small travel-size litter box. We found a big plastic bowl at the thrift store that fits just right in between the front and back seats of the car that works out great for traveling. One thing I have learned by experience is not to take them to the pet area at the rest stops. Number one, they don't understand that they are supposed to potty outside (especially if you have an indoor cat). Number two, you will be buying some kind of flea and tick spray at the next truck stop. And I thought it would be a good idea to get her out of the car for a while…Nope, bad idea!

If your assignment calls for travel on an airplane there are more rules and regulations that go with that adventure. First of all, you want to go to the airline's website and see what their rules are for traveling with a pet. When you make your arrangements, you need to inform the airline that you will have a pet. It is very important to make arrangements for Rover, instead of just showing up with him. Airlines usually charge an extra $75 to $150 for the pet. When making your travel arrangements try to get non-stop flights.

For the airline websites that I visited, most of them required the pet to be in a carrier that can fit underneath the seat in front of you. This carrier is also counted as one of your carry-ons. While on the airplane or in the airport, the pet is not allowed out of that carrier; therefore, remember to take Rover to potty before entering the airport. Look for a pet relief area outside of the airport entrance. There is a list of airports and their pet relief areas at www.petfriendly.com.

One of the easier ways to travel with your pet is in a recreational vehicle (RV). The pet is always at home and doesn't have to get used to a new apartment every three to six months, just like their owners.

You still have to make sure that the RV park you are staying in is pet friendly, but most of them that I have been in are pet friendly. There may be some breed restrictions, but the size restrictions are not as strict as they are in an apartment. Keep in mind that most RV parks do not allow you to leave a dog unattended in the RV all day while you are at work related to the health risk of your pet.

Along with their leash and their favorite toy, you may want to get an exercise cage. There are all kinds of exercise cages, and most of them fold down. Of course, if you have a larger dog, you will want to take them for walks more often. I've seen a few traveling cats in my travels. Most of them are indoor cats, but I know a few who have cats that can be let outside and will come back to the RV. Most felines that I have been around though usually don't adjust to new places as well as a canine.

As with a new apartment, you want to make sure that there are no dangers for your pet. Make sure that cords can't be played with and cleaning materials are safely tucked under the cabinets, along with all the bug sprays. As with household furniture, you may also want to cover your furniture with a sheet or rug. I saw one RV where they had made seat covers out of rugs found at a thrift store.

If you have a bumper pull of 5th wheel, you would want your pet to ride in the truck with you. If you have a motorhome, the same rules apply for cars in that they either need to be crated or seat-belted/harnessed in. Once again, in case of an accident, you don't want Rover to go flying.

Here are a few more questions and answers about pets!

~*~

The last dog that I owned was a Pomeranian/Chihuahua mix. She was a little dog with a big attitude. Any suggestions on reducing the amount of barking?

"I think small dogs tend to have more attitude." It's a common joke. It's funny to consider that small dogs have the Napoleon complex. Larger dogs seem to be much quieter and more secure than smaller breeds. They also seem to do less damage to property than small breed dogs can do. I think that owners let them get away with being loud or aggressive simply because they are so small. Everyone laughs at them and thinks it's "cute" when they get tough. People are never afraid of them. If a dog weighing 80 pounds acted the same way, they would be locked up, given up for adoption, or fenced all the time, etc. They would not enjoy the same freedom.

I have had several experiences training small dogs (when pet sitting for friends). It takes me about 4 days to break the barking habit. But, when they return to their owners, the habit starts again. This is usually because the owners put up with it. They think, "It's annoying, but not dangerous, so let's just ignore it." The problem is that when your dog constantly barks they are not at peace and are not well adjusted. They are anxious and nervous. Not happy campers!

The good news: it's very easy to break the habit (and who wants to travel alone? Don't you want your friend with you?) It only takes consistency. Every time he barks, give him a sharp and loud "no." You might be saying "no" every 12 seconds for a few days, but eventually he should understand. Don't let them bark when you enter the house. Don't let them bark when the doorbell rings. Don't let them bark at anything. If you start to let it slide and they get away with it a few times you are defeating the purpose.

Dogs are simple creatures; they don't understand "sometimes" or "maybe." They only understand absolute "yes" and "no." So be consistent, be in charge, be the pack leader, command respect. When you do this, your dog will feel better adjusted and will gain more freedom. Ceaser the "Dog Whisperer" has taught us more about dogs than we ever understood. But you must implement his ideas for them to be effective, not just listen to admire them.

Besides their usual yearly rabies shot, what other pet health needs do traveling pet owners need to be aware of?

In my opinion, heartworm, flea, and tick control are the most important preventative measures a pet owner can take. Fleas transmit tapeworm and cause flea allergy dermatitis. Ticks spread spotted fever, Lyme disease, and many other diseases. Heartworms, which are transmitted by mosquitoes, can cause liver failure, damage to the heart, lungs, and other organs, and many other serious health problems. Heartworm disease may even kill your pet. Heartworm, flea, and tick prevention is important, regardless of whether or not you are traveling. It can be even more important when you are on the road because you could be exposing your animal to different risk levels of these parasites in different areas of the country. It is so easy and inexpensive to have these preventative measures taken to protect your pet's health.

What do you do with your pets if you have to leave for a long period of time and are unable to take the pets?

When we travel for short vacations, we try our hardest to find accommodations for them to join us. However, when this is not possible, we find local resources for pet sitting. We usually start this process as soon as we arrive at a new location. We ask for local recommendations from co-workers that have pets, neighbors, or other dog owners that we meet. We also use Craigslist and Google to locate companies and individuals in our area that provide pet services. If we decide to use a pet sitter from Craigslist or Google, we always arrange to meet them ahead of time and we check their references.

How do you find a reputable veterinarian once you get to your destination?

We usually will go to a veterinarian that is close to home. This way, if trouble arises with one of our dogs, we are close and can get them there as soon as possible. If you don't trust the vets close to your new home, I would get some recommendations from co-workers, neighbors, or friends. Yelp.com is also a great resource to find out what other pet owners are saying about your local vet clinics.

Any tips on reducing the anxiety of a move with pets?

Yes. First, make sure your pet can handle a long trip in the car. Condition the pets to small or short moves and they will accommodate the change over time. They actually adapt much faster than humans do. Simple minds only require simple things to make them happy, unlike most humans! Some animals have more anxiety than others in the car. It is best to address any anxiety disorders before you get on the road. Also, as soon as you move into your new place, set up a comfy and familiar bed and toy in a quiet area (if possible) for your dog or cat while you unload and unpack. Sometimes moving your stuff in and out of different homes can be stressful. This is a way to keep him calm by surrounding him with familiar scents in your new place.

How do I make sure my pet has enough, but not too much, food?

This is something that your veterinarian can help you determine. Your pet's food intake can be determined by its weight, activity level, health conditions, etc. Unlike humans, pets usually cannot feed themselves. If they are over or underweight, it's almost always the owner's problem. Please be responsible and feed your pet in a healthy manner.

What helpful hints would have for owners of bigger dogs?

Sometimes larger dogs get a bad rap. Make sure that your larger dog is well adjusted. This means that he does not show aggressive behavior, does not bark uncontrollably, and is not easily stressed. You may need to address behavior issues with training before traveling. Housing is sometimes a little more challenging with larger animals, so if your dog can prove that it is well behaved, their size can be overlooked.

Chapter Eighteen

Traveling In An RV

A journey is a person in itself; no two are alike. And all plans, safeguards, policing, and coercion are fruitless. We find that after years of struggle that we do not take a trip; a trip takes us. (John Steinbeck)

Making The Decision To Travel In An RV

Whether I was in Oklahoma, Mississippi, California, or Iowa, I have always had the same accommodation—a twenty-nine foot travel trailer. Not exactly luxurious accommodations, but at least I didn't have to pack and unpack every three to six months. No, this lifestyle is not for everyone, but for me and my family it was just perfect.

It all started after my first assignment. Moving into the apartment in Phoenix was okay for the three of us, until we went to move out. Our home was two hundred miles away from the assignment and we found ourselves taking more and more stuff down each time we returned to the Phoenix apartment from our home in Lake Havasu City, Arizona.

After taking two trips with a U-Haul trailer to get everything back, we decided that we didn't adjust very well to keeping it downsized at the apartment. With the three of us, we needed to either buy a bigger permanent hauling trailer or look at a travel trailer.

Off to California I went, while my son and husband stayed back in Arizona to gather up some loose ends before joining me. I was by myself for one month, living in a motel room, since housing was scarce related to seasonal workers. After the family joined me, we moved into a larger motel suite, but that quickly became too close for comfort, hence the search for the alternative of a recreational vehicle (RV).

One thing that I'm frequently asked is, "Is there always a campground near the hospital?" Well, that it where planning takes effect. The first thing that I check out when my recruiter mentions an assignment to me is where the nearest RV park is located. The most I've ever had to drive is 20 minutes to the hospital from the RV park. The most common places to look for a campground are www.woodalls.com, www.goodsamclub.com, and www.rvparkreviews.com With more and more nurses choosing the RV housing option, more and more travel companies housing departments and/or recruiters will assist you in finding a local campground.

What Type To Look For

What exactly people are looking for in an RV and their needs are so diverse that companies have been expanding their floor plans on a yearly basis. We started our hunt for an RV by visiting as many dealers as we could find in central California. When you go, be sure to also ask about any RV shows that might be coming up in the area.

After you have been to a few dealers, make a list of exactly what you want in an RV. Also, when you are out browsing, look at several different types of RVs. Most full-timers are either in a Class A Motorhome or 5th Wheel, but some prefer to travel in a travel trailer (bumper pull) or Class C Motorhome (a smaller vehicle like a Minnie Winnie).

The least expensive of these options is a travel trailer. A good one will average $15K to $35K, depending on size. If you are full-timing by yourself, you really need to consider one that is 25 ft. in length. If there are two of you, I would consider a 30 foot model. If you have children, look at one with a bunk system in the back. In my travels, I have seen families with four children traveling full time in a four-bunk travel trailer; therefore, this might be a perfect option instead of trying to find a larger apartment. We had a thirty-six footer that seemed to be just right for our family of three. It had two bedrooms so everyone could still have some sense of privacy.

Your next option, price-wise, would be a fifth wheel. These are generally priced from $30K to $110K on the new market. According to a friend of mind, those are much easier to handle than a bumper-pulled travel trailer and easier to hook/unhook from your vehicle.

In Arkansas I came across a travel nurse who was living in a Class C Motorhome. Those are the smaller motorhomes that are usually easily recognized by the over-the-cab bed or storage. This traveler only had his wife and dog with him. In the last year, I have seen a significant rise in the use of Class C's by single women related to the fact that they are not as intimidated as the bigger Class A's. The cost of a Class C runs on average $60K to $135K. They come in many variations now, including with slide-out and storage compartments instead of a bed over-the-cab.

This type of home might be looked at by a family of four, with the option of the over-cab-queen size bed for the parents and twin beds in the back for the children. I could definitely picture myself in one of these if I were a single female. Instead of having to get out for sleeping or using the restroom while on the road, you can just pull over and go to the back and leave the doors locked.

The largest and most expensive option would be a Class A Motorhome, which are the ones that are "bus"-sized. These range in price from $80K to over a million dollars. Nice and spacious, they are definitely homes-away-from-home! Your gasoline Class As are the least expensive options, but they also have the lowest resale value. The diesel Class As are more expensive, but they hold more of their value when it comes time for a resale.

Coming in a wide variety, many are from 35 ft. to 40 ft. on the average; these babies come packed not only with a kitchen sink, but also a dishwasher as an option. After taking a tour of a factory in Iowa, I ventured into an RV that not only had a flat screen television, but also a complete entertainment system, including a fireplace. Now *that* is what I call entertainment!

Basic Buying Guide

Take a look at many floor plans. Where are the beds and the kitchen? We have found, in buying a travel trailer, that it is easier when stopping along the way if the bed is in the back. This way you can load up the kitchen/living area in the front of the trailer, with the bath in the middle. This way you can have all the extra weight in the front and you don't have to load and unload all the extras every time. All that is required is to open up the back door and crawl into the bed.

If you have a motorhome, make sure that you have a path from the front of the rig to the back where your bed is, or when on the road use the fold-out couch in the front of the coach and store all the extra stuff in the back. This, of course, will all depend on how many "extra" goodies you have along with you. We carried an extra outdoor table and chairs, plus at one time I had my outdoor barrel pond. The less you carry, the better off you are, but as any traveler can tell you, it is always easier said than done.

With any travel trailer or 5th wheel, the first thing you need to know is how much weight your tow vehicle can handle. In your operator's guide you will find the towing capacity. Tell the dealer, the first thing, what type of vehicle you are using for a tow vehicle, what type of tow package (extra transmission cooler and gauges), and any special items you might have on the vehicle that would affect its towing capacity. For example, our truck will pull 9500 lbs.; we have an external and internal transmission cooler, extra transmission gauges, and air suspension.

Once you know the amount that your vehicle can pull, you want to look for a trailer that is about 70% of that weight. Therefore, the trailer that I would be looking for would be approximately 6650 lbs. Once you have added all your living supplies, the trailer should weigh no more than 80% of your towing capacity. If, for some reason, you go over your 100% towing capacity and you get into an accident, you have a good chance of being liable due to the fact that your weight limit exceeds what your vehicle can handle.

Make sure that you have the proper hitch, also. You not only need the proper size ball hitch, but you need the appropriate weight distribution bar, anti-sway bar, and get the best brake control system that you can afford. Skimping on these details can make a big difference if you get into high winds, going up and down steep grades, or in case you need to make an emergency stop.

A big thing for full-timers is storage! Make sure that you have enough storage. This is where the motorhomes have a great advantage over a travel trailer. The "basement" storage is a great plus. There is also more closet space in the motorhomes than in a travel trailer on the average, although I have been in a few 5th wheels that have quite a bit of closet space. If you have a handyman around, an option for a travel trailer would be to convert a bunk system in a travel trailer to more closet space. One trailer I looked at last year in a home show had a small slide-out in the back where the kids had their own couch and entertainment center, along with fold up bunks. In my situation, it would be so easy to take out the bunks and make a closet out of that and use the small slide-out for an office space. When we were looking at toy-haulers once, a dealer told us about a full-timer who couldn't find exactly what she needed, so she took an empty trailer and put in her own furniture to make a home-on-wheels. In other words, use your imagination when you go shopping!

A few other things to consider when shopping are the bedroom and bathroom. Lie on the bed and see how it feels. Some aren't the most comfortable beds, but can be made more manageable by putting one of those space-age technology types of foam mattresses over it. In the last few years I have seen more and more motorhomes with the sleep number bed system as an option. You can also purchase a sleep number bed mattress system at your local camping supply store.

Sit on the commode and see if there is enough leg and arm space. The last few years I have seen more and more RVs with the optional shower on one side and the commode on the other side. What size shower and/or tub do you need? We were very lucky in the fact that we had a full-size tub. There wasn't too much difference between the tub size in my permanent home and my RV. Some have half-tubs and some just have the shower. This last year I even saw one that had a whirlpool tub in it, although that motorhome was a little more expensive than I could afford at $350K.

Also, look at what type of electrical system it has. The standard RV has either 30 amp or 50 amp, unless you get a gigantic motorhome, which may require 100 amp. With a 30 amp vehicle you might find yourself turning off the air conditioner while you run the microwave or blow-dry your hair. Usually, with a 50 amp, you don't have to worry about that. Also, it will make a big difference if you have one or two air conditioning units. With the RVs that have two air conditioning units, you will need a 50 amp or an upgraded electrical system that can handle all of your power needs.

What Options To Look For

In the beginning of the RV building world there were only two or three floor plans and styles that you could choose from, but now the options are almost endless.

In the travel trailer world you can find trailers with garages, trailers that have "toy boxes" for your motorcycles or golf cart, ones with slide-outs, and trailers with utility closets in the back.

In Arizona and Southern California, the toy haulers are quite common. Not only do people haul around their dune buggies and four wheelers, but golf carts and small electric cars. With gas prices soaring ever so high, I have often thought about getting a toy hauler and an electric car. I have also heard that some toy hauler can handle a smart car.

The smaller garages at the back would also be nice for a full-timer. You could store things that you might use seasonally or keep your bikes locked up. The other day we saw an RV with a small storage area in the whole back of the trailer that opened up and you could hang items like your hoses, utility equipment, and miscellaneous hardware in there.

Other options that you may look for in the kitchen are a full-size or four-door refrigerator and freezer with an icemaker. These are great and can be found in a lot of the newer motorhomes. Also, in the kitchens of the newer motorhomes you might find a dishwasher or a trash compactor.

In many of the 5th wheels and motorhomes you might find a combination washer and dryer. Although these are very small, they are great to use for everyday clothes. You will probably still want to use the bigger machines at the laundromat for your bigger items, such as towels and linens.

In the living room area you can look for such options as an electric fireplace, entertainment center, computer center and satellite dish. Satellite dishes also come in many types, from just plain old television to ones that will also help you get onto the Internet and even track while moving (this will be discussed later on in more depth).

To make traveling and maneuvering easier you can find motorhomes with a navigational system and cameras in the back of the rig to assist you in backing up. After you have had either of these for very long you will wonder how you ever lived without them! I can't imagine going anywhere without my navigational system.

Motorhomes usually come with some kind of basement storage. This is the one major advantage to having a larger motorhome; there is a lot more storage for full-timers! There is even one company who not only makes a basement but also has an upstairs. That's right, a set of stairs leads you to the top of the RV where there is a patio set up with grill, tables, chairs, and an umbrella. Of course you would want to take the umbrella down while you're going down the road.

There are many, many other options that you can have. What you have to decide is which options are worth the money for you and your family.

Internet Access While On The Road

Most RV parks now have wireless access. In fact, I searched all the campgrounds that we had stayed at and they all had wireless access. Some are free and some require an additional fee. All you need is a wireless card, which most computers come with now. You just look for a signal then type in your user name and password if needed. The most important thing you want to remember when hooking into an open wireless service is that you make sure that the type of connection you make is public. By choosing this option, discovery of other computers and devices on the network will be limited, and the use of the network by some programs might be restricted. We also have a signal booster that takes the wireless signals and increases the strength to a tolerable level.

Another option is through your cell phone. There are two ways to do this. Most commonly used is making your cell phone a "hot spot" and getting wireless Internet for your phone. Depending on the packages, you will really have to watch your time and gigs used. Going over the allotted amount can cost you hundreds of dollars. Or, for about $20, you can purchase a cable that will connect your cell phone to your computer through the USB port. After purchasing a dialup program for another $20, you can then use your phone. Check with your cell phone carrier about charges for this service. Some companies take air time out of your minutes, while others will let you use it unlimited for a set price.

Wireless cards are also an option. These cards are offered through cell phone companies and are like a wireless system that you plug into the network port on your laptop. In the bigger cities you can have up to broadband speeds with these systems, although the current price is about $60/month.

For your own personal broadband network you can also do the satellite Internet. There are three types that you can get. The first is a dish that is set up on a tripod. Every time you go to a new place, you set up the tripod and dish, aim the satellite, and you're off and running. The first couple of times you try it can be frustrating, but after much perseverance, you can do it! After our 3rd assignment and using this, I could get things set up in about 20 minutes.

Another system is on top of the rig, and you still have to manually adjust it every time. This really isn't too bad if you are moving only once every three to six months and can be easily figured out as with the tripod system. The disadvantage to this is that you have to make sure that your rig is perfectly level or you won't be able to find the satellite connection.

The least work that you will have to do is with an automatic satellite, but it is much more expensive than the first two. In fact, in 2004, we paid $1,500 for our system on the tripod, while a friend of mine paid $5,000 for her automatic one on top of the rig. It seems like she has more trouble with her system than I have with my system, and every time there is a problem she has to take her rig into the dealer to have the satellite worked on, where ours is much more easily repaired being that it is not connected to the rig. The system that you choose will depend on how computer savvy you are.

The drawback from having a system like we had is that you either have to be certified to aim the satellite or hire a certified installer to come out and aim the dish every time you move. I would recommend taking the class so you can aim your own dish.

In Conclusion

The mobile lifestyle is one that can be very rewarding if you hate packing and unpacking every few months. If you keep your traveling goodies to a minimum, your home can easily be unhooked from the park and moved in a just a few short hours.

When I first wrote this chapter we were in Iowa with our 35 ft. Dutchman. Coming out of Iowa we had a semi-tractor/trailer pass us and we started fishtailing. Long story short, an hour later the trailer slid onto the tires and we closed down I-35 and I-70 for 30 minutes while they loaded us onto a wrecker.

We went back to traveling in apartments until our misadventures in a motel room in North Dakota (13 weeks with 2 cats and a hubby is a LONG time in one room!).

We now have a 29 ft. Coleman TT and absolutely love it with the duel slides in the living room! The cats love their new room to roam and are totally into the RV lifestyle! They can see out all the windows in the dining room, living room, and kitchen area.

Three years ago, I started a Facebook group for traveling nurses and healthcare professionals who travel in an RV. We have nurses that are in travel trailers, 5th wheels, Class C motorhomes, and Class

A motorhomes. Come on and join us! https://www.facebook.com/groups/HighwayHypodermicsRvTravelers/

The one thing I hear the most is, "I wished I would have gotten an RV a lot sooner!"

Chapter Nineteen

Homeschooling While On The Road

Education begins at home and I applaud the parents who recognize that they, not someone else, must take responsibility to assure that their children are well educated. (Ernest Istook)

For years I thought I couldn't do travel nursing because my son was in public school and I needed to give him a stable environment in which to live. I planned on going into travel nursing the minute he graduated. That was until April 2003.

My son's school informed me that my child had figured out that if he went to this in-school suspension program, he could do his schoolwork in another classroom without all the kids who called him names and picked on him unmercifully because of his size. Kids are just cruel in junior high school, especially if you don't conform to their idea of what a "cool" teenager is.

The counselor told me, "I just don't know what I'm going to do with your son next year." I looked at my husband, who shrugged, and then I turned to the school counselor and advised him that I didn't think that he was going to have to worry about my son next year.

My bachelor's degree actually is not in nursing; it's in secondary science education. After we went home, I informed my husband that I believed that it was time to hit the road. If they didn't know what to do with him, I didn't see where it would harm my child to be on the road fulltime in an "unstable" environment when he could learn things all over the United States.

I had a teacher's certificate at one time (lapsed when I went into nursing), and I didn't see where the school system was doing a better job than I could do at home. My suspicions were confirmed when I did his diagnostic testing and found that my 7th grader was actually functioning at a 3rd to 4th grade level. That made me a real believer in the Individual Educational Program (IEP) that schools have now set forth.

Okay, off of my soapbox and back into the real world of homeschooling. The decision was easy for me, since I had an educational degree background. After this chapter, you will have the knowledge to make an informed decision on whether or not homeschooling is right for you and your children, as well as what alternatives you have.

Exactly What Is Homeschooling?

Homeschooling is getting out the books every morning and doing lessons in math, science, history, grammar, and literature. Homeschooling is taking field trips. Homeschooling is running around in your pajamas doing algebra. Homeschooling is many different things that all surround the idea of teaching your children at home.

First is the traditional style of homeschooling. This follows the standard way of doing schoolwork. With this style, you find books that are geared towards the age and grade of your child and you have traditional reading, worksheets, and then tests. There are several curriculums that you can use for this style, including Alpha Omega Lifepacs (which use workbooks) or textbooks through Abeka Publishing or Bob Jones Publishing, which are Christian-based curriculums. There is a giant list of resources at www.homeschool.com/resources/. I am not familiar with all the companies or all the textbooks, but this is a great place to start your search for the best program that will fit your situation.

Another great source is to find out what the schools do with their old books. I found a gold mine of used schoolbooks in Oklahoma City. I also purchased a book with a plethora of resources called, "The Complete Home Learning Source Book." Check with your local Homeschool Association and find out when and where the next book fair is going to be. You can also get an idea of what other parents are using before you set out on your travel nursing adventure.

Computer learning is next on the list. Through some programs called "Switched On Schoolhouse" or the "Robinson Curriculum," you install the program onto your computer and your child's computer and you have control over the student's curriculum. This is a great way to do things for some children and teachers alike. The lessons are automatically graded, and learning is on an interactive level.

Computer learning can also be accomplished with some programs online in which you enroll your child in a school, and they take classes online with teachers and tests through the Internet. This is a great option for the parent who is uneasy about attempting to teach their child at home. www.k12.com offers a directory of online public schools, online private schools, and individual courses.

Unit studies are very popular also. This is where you teach your children all subjects that are on one subject. This can be very useful as a traveling nurse, because you can do unit studies on the state in which you are traveling as well as the surrounding states. Children are taught math, as in how much is needed to purchase groceries, history through the state sites, biology through seeing what grows in that area and what type of energy is most common there, and are there any windmills or hydro plants? You can view guides for unit studies at www.homeschoollearning.com. By doing a search online you can find free unit study guides.

The new out-of-the-box type of homeschooling is called "un-schooling." This is where the children learn from day-to-day events. No, this does not mean that they sit and watch television and play video games all day, but things are learned from experiences. Parents will often spend time going through the newspaper with their children and learning what is going on in the world and why things are happening the way they are. Math is learned from figuring out how much things cost, how to budget, and other word problems. Science is learned by exploring a park and checking out all the leaves and grasses and attempting to identify what kind of things are in the environment. No tests are done, but the children learn by experience. I think this is a great way of learning for travel nurses to incorporate, at least part-time, since we travel so much and see so many different things and live in so many different cultures.

All these curriculums can be found by doing a search online, contacting the publishing houses, and on eBay. If you are interested in looking at sources in your community, find your local homeschool association and ask for their help in finding homeschool materials. Materials can also be found at general bookstores. Even Borders, Barnes and Noble, and Hastings can special order books for you.

Personally, I buy my books online at PennywiseLearning.com or on eBay. After my son had completed all his material on another sheet of paper or in his notebook, I then sold the material as used on eBay and recovered at least half of the money that I had spent to get the books.

What About State Laws?

Laws are different in each state. As a traveling nurse, you primarily have to go by what your home state laws are, but there are certain situations when you will have to abide by the state laws to which you are assigned.

For instance, in Mississippi they have a law that states all recreational vehicle parks have to have documentation that your child, who is running around during the day, actually is homeschooled. For this, I just gave the park manager a copy of the affidavit that I had filled out for my home state, affirming that my child was homeschooled. This may also mean getting a letter from the school district in states that require you to keep in touch with the school district.

When we were in Tennessee, we didn't have to have a letter for the apartment complex, but we did need to have a letter for my 17-year-old's place of employment from the school board, stating that our son was enrolled in homeschool. To accomplish this, I wrote a letter of intent to the school board here and sent them verification of my qualifications to teach, and they sent me a letter for my son's employer that stated he was in homeschool. It was then I realized that in some states you must have a copy of your bachelor's degree in order to teach high school.

Why did I have to go through all of this? Because in different states you have different age requirements on how long your children must attend school. Although we were okay with our home state of Idaho, we still had to comply with some of the state requirements because of housing and employment. There are other states that we have been in (Oklahoma, Florida, California, and Iowa) where we were not required to do anything special related to our home residence, since it was not in those states. If there is a problem, someone will tell you; until that time it is usually best just to cruise through your assignment following your home state's rules.

Finding out the laws in each state is not as difficult as you would think; all you need to do is bookmark on your computer www.hslda.org. If you do not have a computer, the information can also be found through that state's department of education or local school district.

Some of the state laws are very restrictive and some are not so restrictive. For example, in Idaho the only rules are that if your child is between the ages of 7 years and 15 you must have some kind of alternative educational program. That means that once children are 16 they can "drop out" of school, although it is not necessarily advised. Other less restrictive states that I have been in are Texas and Oklahoma.

Medium restrictive states that I have been in include Arizona, California, and Mississippi. These states require such things as filing an annual affidavit or letter of intent, maintaining attendance records, and requiring basic subjects such as math, science, history, grammar, and literature. Tennessee also requires that you must have a college education to teach high school and that your child has to attend school until they are 18.

Other more restrictive states require you to have more extensive subjects, such as algebra, geometry, physics, and chemistry, along with documentation of the hours spent in school, days spent in school, maintaining accurate records, and taking state-wide standardized tests.

Other good resources for homeschool information include: www.homeschoolacademy.com, www.time4learning.com, www.saxonhomeschool.hmhco.com, and www.discoveryeducation.com.

Driving Me Crazy

Literally, for a homeschooled child of a traveling nurse, I was literally nuts by the time we wove our way through all the legal mumble jumble, but we made it.

Driver's education at our house was done by the "principal"—i.e. Dad! If you are located in a heavily populated area, I would suggest that you find a good driving school. If you are in a rural area, good old country roads that are unpopulated provide a good start. Talk to other nurses to see if someone has a place out in the country for a "feel" of what it is like to drive for the first time. Of course this is only done after your child has a learning permit.

Getting the learning permit—*that* was what drove me crazy with all these state rules. It is always best to have your child take the test in the state in which you are a resident, but if you are across the country and you think that your child is ready, then it can be done in some states. The key to this is that hopefully you are in a state in which your son/daughter can be a resident of that state, and you do not have to be. This is easily accomplished if your child has some kind of employment.

For instance, at the time we still had the RV and my son worked for the campground part-time. It wasn't much, but it did give him a paycheck. We used a national bank, separate from our bank, and used his address as the assignment address. Sonny has a job and a bank account, now he can pass for a resident—well, at least in some states.

There are other states in which the parents also have to have a driver's license in that state. Although not advisable, if need be, your spouse can get a driver's license in the new state, but do not ever get your driver's license in another state, because then you are going to have trouble with the Internal Revenue Service in establishing a tax home. It's not going to look good with your spouse being a resident of another state, but it is just one option to consider.

As previously stated, if at all possible find a local driving school for your child; if one can not be found, there are lots of driver's programs online, such as the one found at www.driversed.com. After completing the program, your child will receive a certificate of completion, which is approved by almost all the states (verify before you begin if you wish). It is a great course that I would recommend to anybody homeschooling their child.

Also, contact your insurance agency and see if they have programs available. We watched a movie and filled out a driving log to receive a discount on our insurance; you can also have your child take the SAT or ACT test and get a reduced "good student" rate. In fact, we kept a travel log for a while after my son completed his regular program in case we needed to prove how many hours he had behind the wheel.

One of the funniest experiences with this whole deal was that when we moved assignments, my son went to apply for his regular permit instead of a learner's permit and they wanted to know if he had any experience with a certified driving instructor. Of course he hadn't, but we had made a trip between assignments back home so he had driven most of the way from Iowa home to Idaho and to Florida. Over 3000 miles and none of it counted because he wasn't with a certified driving instructor.

What About Socialization?

You know what is funny about people who ask this question? They will also tell you about the terrible things that happened at Columbine High School, the Sandy Hook Elementary shootings, and all the teens that are arrested at school for having guns in their possession. Why did all these bad things happen at school? Because the majority of teens think that to be cool you have to knock someone else's "coolness" down. Unless your child is perfect, chances are they are being teased or bullied at school by someone. That is what I call "great socialization!"

At one of the RV parks we were in, the owner and manager said that the children were not allowed to use the recreational equipment on the weekends when other children were there, but they had found that the homeschooled children were much better behaved and they could go over there any time if it was just them. Several times I had people come to my trailer and ask if "the boy over there is your son?" After answering, "Yes," they would proceed to tell me what good things my son had done and then ask, "Is he homeschooled?" I don't know what other proof you need, but my personal experience is that people can tell by your child's behavior that they are homeschooled.

Yes, I believe our children need to be around other children of the same age, but with the proper influence. After getting settled into an area, we start the search for a church that has a good group of teenagers. I am a member of the Nazarene Church, and my husband was born and raised Baptist; therefore, we tend to stick to one of those two denominations. But there was one assignment in which we were Lutherans, related to the fact that that was where the best group of teenagers for our son to be social with.

Other than church groups, there are many other groups such as Boy Scouts, Girl Scouts, and Explorer Groups. Look for groups such as a bowling league, baseball league, basketball league, or the YMCA. The local Chamber of Commerce or Parks and Recreation Departments at the city should be able to help you in choosing a place for your child to interact with other children. Also, look for information through the local homeschool association.

From A Child

As a writing assignment in 2006, I asked my son, Kalen (17 y/o at that time), what he would like to tell others about his life as the son of a fulltime traveling nurse, and this is what he had to say.

"I love traveling with my parents because I get to see so many exciting places. When I was in Arizona, I got to see the Grand Canyon, and I have been to an old gold mine. I got to go to the London Bridge on several occasions. In 2001, my family and I went several times to Chase Stadium, which was known back then as Bank One Ballpark, in Phoenix, to see the Diamondbacks play. This is also the year they won the World Series.

When I was in California I got to do several things, including learning a little Spanish, going to Monterey to go deep-sea fishing in the Pacific Ocean, and I even got to experience my first earthquake.

When we went to Iowa, I got my first job at a restaurant near the lake. Mom and I also got to go to see the scene of the crash where Buddy Holly, the Big Bopper, and Ritchie Valens passed away, which is now known as 'the day that the music died.'

When I went to Oklahoma, I was in Oklahoma City. I got to go to the Oklahoma Bombing site. Although I was living in Oklahoma at the time of the bombing, I don't remember much of it, so it was great to learn about something that happened while I was an Okie. In Tulsa we went to see the Tulsa Drillers, which is a AAA baseball team. I met a few friends there also. We also went to Tulsa to get my 16th birthday present, a 1985 Ford Mustang convertible, which my uncle painted for me.

Our fifth assignment was in Mississippi. I got to go to Corinth, where the north and south train route met with the east to west train at the crossroads. I got to visit several battlefields, but the most memorable one was the site of the Battle of Shiloh.

Next we went to Florida. While I was there, I worked for a local newspaper and then started my fast food career. Hurricane Wilma came to visit us, and that was a totally different experience for me! There was so much devastation in Florida that I can't imagine what it was like for those who were in Hurricane Katrina.

Unfortunately, my Mustang didn't make it out of Florida. When I was driving from Fort Lauderdale, Florida, to Nashville, Tennessee, the engine gave it up on the side of the road. I will just have to wait until the next assignment to think about another vehicle.

Right now I'm in Tennessee. I have made a great career choice here. I love my fast food job, and have even been recommended for a managerial position when I turn 18 years old. I have always wanted to be a police officer, but I am currently thinking about going into restaurant management instead.

Although I have had some great adventures over the last three years, there have been some drawbacks. Seems like every time that I get settled into a job and a new store, then it's time to move again. I have a long list of friends, but I don't see them. Most of my friends don't come from school, but from the church youth groups that I attend while on the road. I also miss my friends in my old hometown of Lake Havasu City, Arizona.

I also met my girlfriend on the road through the Internet. I haven't got to meet her yet, but my mom says that she is going to take an assignment in Washington this next year so that we can meet "in reality." This may seem strange to some teens, but hey, my mom and step-dad met that way! We have been chatting on the phone and computer for almost two years now. I have learned so much more traveling than I ever could learn in a classroom. I would definitely recommend nurses taking their children with them if at all possible. I love my life on the road! Thanks, Mom!"

Update 2017: Kalen has been living in Washington since my assignment there in 2006. In those 11 years, his girlfriend is now his wife, and they are the proud parents of Tia and Buddy, my grand-dogs.

In Conclusion

No, homeschooling is not for every parent on the road, but I have had several nurses ask me exactly how I homeschool my child, how I started out, and the benefits that I have found since we're on the road fulltime.

Yes, there are other ways to provide school for children while on the road, such as switching assignments in the middle of semesters, at Christmas break, or during summer break. You can get in three good assignments this way. Others that I know take a nine-month assignment during the school year, and then take a summer assignment somewhere in the cooler north or on the beach. Other parents choose to stay within a few hundred miles of their families, and their families stay at home. There is no *one* right or wrong way to school your child while on the road. You have to do what is most comfortable for you and your family.

For those of you who choose to homeschool, the freedom of learning live historical facts is worth "dragging" your children around the United States. I have absolutely no doubt that it makes them better students for the future, and I hope that this chapter will give you the motivation that you need to make that leap into the future of homeschooling.

Chapter Twenty
On The Road Again With the Gang

"On the road again, I just can't wait to get on the road again." (Willie Nelson)

~*~

Heather from Wisconsin

Heather is a wound/ostomy/continence/ortho nurse from Wisconsin who travels for the location and a great recruiter. She takes the housing stipend and finds her own housing. She has been a traveler for almost a year with RN Network. Her favorite city to work with has been Viroqua, WI.

About her first travel assignment she writes, "Walking into the first day, first travel job. AMAZING. This hospital was a high traveler facility. I found out why pretty quick. But, I didn't let that bother me, and did everything in my power to take care of my patients, to learn quickly and just plain be open. The best thing I feel I ever did, and will always carry with me is to be positive. No matter what the staffing complains about regarding their docs, their facility, be positive. If there were negative comments, I would try and turn it around by comparing to other facilities having the same problems, they are not the only ones and if they can always remember the patient is first and make them think about why they went into nursing in the first place, they could get through anything as a team for the patient! It always worked!"

She would like share with other travelers, "Go in positive, every single day. Don't get into their negativity regarding the facility or coworkers, even if you agree. Just like the military, make sure it is written in the contract, not just a "verbal handshake" it doesn't work that way, anywhere."

~*~

Nina from North Carolina

Nina is an OR nurse from North Carolina who travels for the location and money. She prefers the travel company stipend to find her own housing. She has been traveling for 2 years and is currently with Soliant Healthcare. Her favorite city has been Morehead City, NC, with her least favorite being Dillon, SC.

About her first assignment she writes, "I arrived on my first travel assignment in Dillon SC on a Sunday afternoon. My company had put me up in a horrible motel I refused to stay in for safety reasons. They had no idea of what was available in the town and did no research. I had to find another place to stay and called them to take care of the bill. We (me, my dog and my cat) stayed in another hotel for a week and then had to leave due to bedbugs. I then stayed in a nicer hotel for a couple of days but couldn't remain because it was 30 minutes away and I had to take call. I checked in to a different motel in the town and was intimidated and threatened so I left; my dog was barking in our room and drug dealing was going on in the motel. We stayed there for only a few hours. Finally, I found an OK hotel for a day. Keep in mind I had been working at the hospital the whole time this went on. During that time one of my colleagues found a realtor who would rent me a house during my assignment there. My company was willing to pay for it. So I finally was able to settle into a pleasant house in a decent neighborhood, but I seriously considered packing up and going home."

She would like to tell other travelers, "If it sounds too good to be true, it is. Sometimes the best way to find housing is talking to your co-workers at the facility. Some recruiters will not back you. Write them off and move on. There are plenty of jobs and plenty of companies. I have worked with several. Don't get discouraged… that's the main thing. I've been in some tough situations and I'm still traveling."

~*~

Erik from South Carolina

Erik is an ER nurse who travels for the money and location. He has been with Supplemental Healthcare for 2 years. His favorite town has been Brooklyn, NY, with is least favorite being Charleston, SC.

About his first assignment he states, "First travel experience was hard to get. I had to find the hospital that would take someone with less than 2 years' experience and also was a first time traveler. Stamford Hospital in Stamford, CT was that hospital. At first I was nervous because I was out of my familiar zone. I didn't know anyone and I was in a new city. As with all travel assignments the first 2 weeks are usually tough. As the weeks progressed I started really enjoying were I was. There is always going to be someone that is "just a nasty person." It is going to be at every hospital that you go to. There is, however, going to always be people that are going to help you out no matter what. By the end of the assignment I knew that travel nursing was something that I was going to enjoy. Now after traveling for 1.5 years I have been to some great places and then some horrible places. Now working at a hospital on the amazing island of Maui."

He would like to tell a first time traveler, "Always ask questions during your phone interview. This is away to understand what is going on. Also, always get things in writing. It doesn't matter what your recruiter says, it needs to be on paper. Talk to other travelers because we can give the advice needed to get you through the assignment. Also remember, the skies the limit. You can go anywhere that you want, just believe in it."

~*~

Teri from Nebraska

Teri is a med/surg nurse who places her priorities on a great recruiter and excellent location! She has been traveling for 4 years and takes the money to find her own housing. She just returned to Trustaff after a not so good assignment with Titan Medical. Her favorite hospitals have been Eastern New Mexico Medical Center in Roswell New Mexico, with one of her favorite assignment being in Shiprock, NM. She didn't fare so well in Santa Fe, NM or Del Rio, TX.

About her first travel assignment she states, "My first travel assignment I went to St. Louis, MO and had a 13 week contract at St. Louis University Hospital travel friendly I enjoyed the staff at the hospital they worked well as a team the communication between staff made a great difference. I traveled to St. Louis, MO and had a 13 week assignment I enjoyed the experience it was St. Louis University

Hospital learned a great deal from my co-workers and stayed 26 weeks. The company at the time did my housing and it all worked out very well."

When asked what she would tell a new travel nurse, she stated, "My housing was done per my travel agency and it was an extended stay worked out really well. You need to remember they think you make take big money so they try and give you the most needy patients or the most admits don't take it serious you get to leave in 13 weeks and your pay check comes every week. My company Trustaff did a good job."

~*~

Cameron from Texas

Cameron is from Texas who has been traveling for 3 years as an ICU nurse with Aureus Medical after having some problems with PPR. He travels for the great location including Seattle, WA and Tucson, AZ. His least favorite place to travel was Appleton, WI. He also likes a healthy paycheck.

About his first assignment he states, "It was awesome. People were friendly and made great friends and I felt like a part of the team."

What would he like to tell the newbies? "Just jump in and everyone will grow to love you."

~*~

Shannon from Arkansas

Shannon is an ER nurse who has traveled for 3 years for the marvelous locations and great money. She currently takes the housing stipend and finds her own. She currently travels with Travel Nurse across America, but has been known to switch companies including NursesRX. Her favorite location was in Burleson, TX with her least favorite in North Little Rock, AR.

About her first assignment she states, "I went into a downtown Ft Worth ER as a new traveler. I had worked previously in ER for 5 years. This particular hospital had no actual nurse to patient ratio, it had the "pull til full" mentality with no regard for nurse or patient safety. Questions were met with more disdain than answers by other nurses.

I almost called it quits on travel but transferred to Burleson and had a much better experience."

She would like to tell other travelers, "There is a certain level of "hazing" at each facility. You have to be pretty thick skinned to make it through this. Generally, after a month or so, things level out more with staff."

~*~

Labellt from Alabama

Labellt is a Medical-Surgical-Emergency-Psychiatric nurse who travels for the great benefits and excellent paychecks. She takes the housing stipend and finds her own housing. In her 3 years of traveling she did have a disastrous assignment with American Mobile, but now finds herself happy with Jackson Nurse Professions. Her favorite location has been Atlanta, GA.

About her first assignment she writes, "I wanted my first travel experience to be in a nearby state somewhere I could work my shifts and drive home when I was finished. I accomplished that by working at a hospital in Atlanta, Ga. on a 13 week assignment. There was a lot to learn including a new computerized charting system. It was a general medicine unit. The nurse patient ratio was 1:5 to 6. There were about 4 other travelers there. Our charge nurse did not take patients. She was very helpful in getting new patients in the bed and doing charge tasks. The nurses were friendly and helpful. I adjusted well considering that we had only two days of orientation. One night I informed the nurse who was covering me that I would go to lunch and gave her my report. While I was at lunch a lab tech called me some lab results and I informed her that I was at lunch and instructed her to call the results to the charge nurse but she would not take the results so the lab tech called the nursing supervisor and reported the charge nurse for not accepting the information. When I returned from lunch the nurses and unit secretary told me that the charge nurse was upset at me for going to lunch. Near the end of the 13 weeks I noticed the other travelers were saying they had been asked to extend but I had not. I called the travel agency and asked them why I wasn't extended and left message for the unit manager to call me because I wanted to find out if I would be extended but I never heard from the unit manager after leaving numerous messages and my recruiter said that she would find out about the extension but was never given an answer. To this day I still do not know why I wasn't extended. The only thing that I could relate to was the anger the charge nurse had for me about going to lunch and she being reported to the supervisor by lab personnel."

What would she like to tell a first timer? "Be as thorough as possible in your work ethic. Be on time and try to finish your work on time. Don't discuss pay with staff on your unit. Take breaks within the proper time frame. Carefully choose your words when talking to staff. Never raise your voice. Maintain your professionalism with staff and other travelers."

~*~

Larry from Michigan

Larry is an ER nurse who travels for the wonderful money and a great recruiter. He takes the housing stipends and finds his own RV park. He has been traveling for 5 years with Rise Medical Staffing after a not so great adventure with Trustaff. His favorite hospital has been Anchorage, AK after a disaster in Lancaster, CA.

About his first assignment he writes, "Travel nursing is a social experiment in personal flexibility. My first assignment was on the "REZ" in Eagle Butte, SD. The Lakota tribe is there and with that an IHS (Indian Health Services) hospital. It was a small rural facility with all the problems of poverty and substance abuse. What I found there is people do not necessarily have a car, may not have running water, may not maintain housing by replacing broken windows. It seemed normal for the wind to blow into the housing. Those that had work did so on firefighting crews during the summer; they probably do not have a "regular" job. This was shocking to a mid-western man that believed people essentially lived the same. I found the work ethic to be very high among the white population and some of the native. Unemployment was a true social ill among many of the Lakota.

One of my native neighbors came to my RV and asked me to "sew up" her significant other. She reported that he had been staggering around and fell into a knife. It was 10 AM and while they drank beer non-stop generally they had a steady gait. I went to see what I could do. Certainly he had a belly wound that was oozing blood. I could not stop the bleeding with direct pressure and gauze so I took him into the IHS facility. Note: The lack of clotting and danger of hemorrhage is a serious problem when the client has ETOH on board. He told me "this is the fourth time she has stabbed me, I think I need to find a new place to live." That was what I thought had happened so I filled out a report and she had 1 overnight in jail. Two days later, around 1A I am getting called out for "I need to talk to you" by this inebriated native woman. There was no way I was going out! She is "really good with a knife" was going through my mind, and I was not going to cause harm to her through escalation. I called the police and they took her in again. After that she left me alone. I helped her decision as I shot skeet in the field behind the mobile home park.

The moral to this story? (1) People are needy, we get sick, have social dysfunction and sometimes to do things that are illegal, it is normal to make a splash; (2) The standard of living varies greatly around America, electricity, running water, sewer and temperature control are luxuries; (3) The best way to feel the culture is live among those you serve. I would not have understood what Native American culture was until I worked on the reservation; (4) Know your limitations, stay will informed and be nice always to everyone."

~*~

Shana from Kentucky

Shana is a Med/Surg nurse who travels for the money and a great recruiter. She takes the housing stipend and finds her own housing. She has been traveling for a year with Medical Staffing Solutions.

She states, "My first assignment was awesome!! The staff at the hospital were very travel nurse friendly. That made a huge difference. I felt that they gave more than enough orientation too (which was like 2 weeks!). I loved my assignment, loved my fellow employees, and had a wonderful clinical nurse and DON. They really made me feel like I was at home and included me as part of the gang. I was put in charge of the unit several times, and was even orientating new nurses for them at times. They extended my contract several times also. I would work for them any time in the future.

I went through 3 recruiters on my first assignment with this company and that made me nervous at first. However, my third and final recruiter is awesome!! He is there any time I need him, answers my calls promptly, is always asking if there is anything else he can do for me, and seems to truly care if I am happy with my assignment. I really appreciate him and hope to work with him for many years to come.

Overall, I have had a wonderful experience traveling. Do your research and don't go with just any company. Know how things work before you choose a company and talk with a recruiter. Always look at the final contract and make sure things you asked for are in there before you sign it."

~*~

Michelle from Florida

Michelle is an oncology nurse who has been traveling with Jackson Nurse Professionals for the last year for the awesome locations and great money. She takes the housing stipend and goes at finding her own housing. Her favorite city has been Orlando, FL.

About her first assignment, she states, "Started off bumpy when I found out our orientation would start the second week of my assignment, but I would be on my own the first week. Luckily, with helpful and friendly staff, I adjusted quickly to the new environment. Had a great experience with no issues with the hospital, staff, or my travel agency."

She would like to tell other travelers, "If you think "maybe I should bring this with me, I am not sure though"...don't bring it, you likely will not need it."

~*~

Jenn from North Carolina

Jenn is an ICU nurse who travels for the great locations followed by the excellent wages. She has been traveling for 4 years and now works with Fusion Medical Staffing after a disastrous outing with Aureus Medical Group. Her least favorite assignment was with Valley Hospital in Las Vegas, NV, with her favorite assignment at Eastern Idaho Regional Medical Center in Idaho Falls, ID.

About her first assignment, she states, "I was sent to Roswell, NM. It was my first day time position, there were only 2 permanent staff members and no director. I was on a med/surg unit not ICU. I worked 4 days a week. The days at work were rough, but doable. I enjoyed getting out to see different sites and visit different places. That's why I wanted to be a travel nurse, work a little and play a lot!! I learned a lot about my practice and how other hospitals were fitting best practice into their policies."

She should like to remind newbies to, "read your contract, know your contract, print your contract. Don't do anything that you have not been trained to do. Wear skates to work (well, not really but be prepared to hustle)."

~*~

Julie from Arkansas

Julie is a Med/Surg nurse who prefers to have an excellent recruiter along with a great salary. She takes the housing stipend and finds her own RV park. She has been traveling for 7 years. Her current company is Liquid Agents after a nightmare of an assignment with American Mobile. Her favorite city has been Los Angeles, CA with her least favorite being Lawton, OK.

About her first travel assignment, she writes, "As a first time traveler, and knowing NO ONE that traveled at that time, I went with American Mobile. They seemed to be the biggest and best travel company out there at the time. I tend to trust people to a fault and the recruiter did not "watch out" for me. Her interest was with the hospital. She did not inform me that I need to ask for a guarantee on my hours and I was left paying for my own apartment on Hollywood Blvd the last 2 weeks of my contract because I kept getting called off when the census fell in the hospital. It was horrible! I loved the hospital (USC) and learned a lot and I LOVED LA! But the fact that I was basically stranded by the recruiter left a horrible taste in my mouth."

What she would like to tell first timers, "Get a guarantee on your hours!!! Other than that, enjoy every minute; learn as much as you can!"

Chapter Twenty-One

Travel Company Profiles

"Every travel company is the best for someone, but no company is the best for everyone."
(Epstein LaRue, 2016)

Accountable Healthcare Staffing

Accountable Healthcare Staffing provides all types of healthcare providers, including RN, LPN, PT, OT, ST, NP, and PA positions for local and travel staff to all 50 states.

They are a large privately owned company that is run by nurses. With over 30 years in the Healthcare Staffing Industry, they understand the importance of relationships. Their best employees are referral from their current staff. They are run BY nurses, FOR nurses. In fact, their 24-hour clinical nurse liaison currently sits on the Georgia State Board of Nursing. They are both TJC certified and a member of NATHO.

They actually LISTEN to what their nurses want and need. Their recruiters are all very experienced and educated. They are here to find you the best possible package out there.

Accountable is proud to offer you registered nurses positions in all 50 states! With their support system, you'll find it's easy to choose travel nursing. Your recruiter works closely with you to find the right position and provides ongoing support. They also have 24-hour phone service for help with housing or any other issues.

Accountable offers higher than average pay, affordable medical, dental, and vision coverage, and a 401(k). They also provide fully furnished, 100% paid housing. In addition, they offer weekly (not daily for TN) pay and bonuses such as sign-on, referral, extension and annual loyalty. Assignments range from 4–13 weeks with extensions that can last 26 weeks if you choose.

Accountable Healthcare benefits include: Medical insurance through Aetna and Dental/Vision provided by Guardian. Other benefits include: Prudential Life and accidental death insurance, Allstate Short term disability, Allstate Accident insurance, Legal Plan of America.

Optional Benefits May Include: Higher Pay, 100% paid fully furnished housing, basic cable, and optional tax advantage program, Travel reimbursement, Sign-on bonus, Completion Bonus, Loyalty Bonus, 401K plan, Group Health Insurance, Weekly Payroll with optional direct deposit, and State License is required. Accountable Healthcare will reimburse licensure up to a predetermined cost to the candidate upon start of assignment.

For more information you can visit them at 999 Yamato Road Suite 210, Boca Raton, Florida 33431. They can be phoned at: 561-235-7810, or visit their website at: *AHCStaff.com.*

~*~

Advantage Medical Professionals

Advantage Medical Professionals provides assignments for RNs, LPNs, CNAS, RTs, and ORTechs. They are a Louisiana based agency with over 30 years in business and six offices throughout Louisiana and Texas as well as travel opportunities in a variety of states throughout the nation.

They feel that their southern hospitality along with professionalism and respect for their nurses are priority. Not only do they have someone on call 24/7, but they also have a clinical nurse liaison that is available. They pride themselves in doing the best to accommodate their nurses. If the nurse isn't happy with their recruiter, they will immediately place them with another recruiter.

Advantage Medical Professionals is a Joint Commission Certified company that offers blue cross insurance along with direct deposit and many other company discounts.

Part of their philosophy at Advantage Medical Professionals is that they believe in treating their nurses like family. That's why they give the same great service to their nurses as they give to their clients. Advantage Medical Professionals have been in the business since 1984 and have a great reputation. They love their nurses!

For more information you can contact them at 3340 Severn Ave., Suite 320, Metairie, LA 7002. They can also be phoned at 504-456-0073, or visit their website at *AdvantageMedicalProfessionals.com.*

~*~

Atlas Med Staffing

The travel nursing industry has evolved, and Atlas was born out of the evolution. Let's be honest, the old recruiter model is inefficient and no longer represents what you as a professional need.

Nurses are sophisticated consumers. You know how to quickly and effectively research online. When it comes to partnering with a staffing firm, you know how and where to do your research. There is a lot of power in that research, and ultimately it will drive your decision on the agency you partner with.

Only the best recruiters will earn the trust and respect of the nurses that put their heart and soul into their profession. Atlas recruiters have to prove themselves and show they legitimately care about their nurses' career advancement and growth. Atlas is focused on being the very best at matching great people to great facilities. They have worked very hard to build a brand that emphasizes their ability to eliminate the headaches of the job search and provide their traveling nurses with the very best opportunity available. That's the Atlas Difference, "Together we can do amazing things."

Benefits are important, and they don't cut any corners. They offer BC/BS health insurance and pick up 60% of the cost for the nurse. They also offer dental and vision insurance, voluntary term life insurance, disability insurance, 401k with matching at 6 months, a $750 referral bonus, and a generous first assignment completion bonus.

Atlas is a veteran owned, mid-sized company. They have always believed in a flat internal business model. They don't have layers of management sitting in offices collecting big checks, or private equity firm owners only interested in the bottom line. That means better pay for their nurses, more freedom for their recruiters, and a happier work environment for all.

For more information, you can contact them at: 11840 Nicholas St., Suite #215, Omaha, NE 68154. They can be phoned here: 855-884-2360 or visit their website here: *www.atlasmedstaff.com.*

~*~

Aureus Medical Group

Aureus Medical Group offers travel and direct hire career opportunities nationwide for RNs, LPNs, CNAs, Advanced Practice, and Allied Health professionals.

Aureus Medical offers travel and direct hire career opportunities nationwide. Their company is privately-held and family-owned. Although they are large enough to offer many career opportunities throughout the United States, they are small enough to know their travelers and provide excellent customer service.

They take a consultative approach to matching travelers to assignments and really get to know their travelers on a personal level. Their travelers work with a team of recruiters and account managers on every assignment. This team-based approach ensures there is always someone available to answer questions and provides for superior customer service. They also have a 24/7 emergency number. They have several RNs on staff as Clinical Nurses. These nurses are available during business hours but are also on-call if an emergency arises. Aureus Medical's Healthcare Staffing Services are certified by the Joint Commission. They are also a member of NATHO.

Unlike other staffing agencies, their travelers work with a team of people on each assignment. Although they will always have a recruiter who will remain their primary contact, they will also work with account managers who are specialized by geographic location as they move from assignment to assignment. This approach allows the traveler to get to know many staffing professionals within the organization and for many staffing professionals to get to know the traveler. If a traveler would prefer to switch recruiters, that option is always available.

Aureus Medical offers a comprehensive benefits package including medical (United Healthcare), dental (Delta Dental), and life (Cigna) insurance coverage. They also offer a 401k plan with matching funds for travelers once they work 3 months and 250 hours. The company matches 100% of the first 3% of traveler contribution, 50% of the next 2%, and 100% of the next 1%. Proceeds are immediately vested at 100%.

Aureus Medical offers an industry-leading "Live & Learn" Tuition

Reimbursement Program which covers the cost of tuition and books, up to $12,000 per degree for bachelor's or master's degrees in Nursing, Allied Health, Healthcare Administration, or Healthcare Education. They also offer paid vacation time, direct deposit, and referral bonuses of up to $1000. In addition, they offer paid private housing through an in-house housing division and travel arrangements through their in-house travel agency.

They have been working in the staffing industry for more than 45 years and they have been staffing medical professionals for more than 30 years. Their recruiters and account managers are dedicated by modality/specialty as well as by geographic location so you can rest assured that there will always be an expert working on your behalf. They have relationships with the top facilities in the country and they work closely with their travelers to make sure each assignment matches their personal and professional goals.

Their mission is to "be the staffing provider and employer of choice by helping people and companies achieve their goals" and they are committed to upholding that mission with the highest level of ethics and integrity. One of the core values of their company is community service and they dedicate thousands of hours and dollars to making their communities better places to live and work.

Aureus Medical is a family-owned and operated company and they treat their travelers like one of the family.

For more information contact them at: 13609 California Street, Omaha, NE 68154. You can phone them at 800-856-5457. Their website can be found at *www.aureusmedical.com.*

~*~

Cirrus Medical Staffing

Cirrus Medical Staffing is an award winning Joint Commission certified healthcare staffing company specializing in the placement of RNs, LPNs, CSTs, and other allied modalities in travel and permanent positions nationwide.

Cirrus Medical Staffing's goal is to create long-term relationships with their travelers. Many of them have been with the company for several years. Their biggest focus is to not only find new travelers to build rapport with but to retain them and build long-term partnerships.

The biggest difference between Cirrus Medical Staffing and other companies is that they customize their compensation package to meet the travel RNs needs and goals. The recruitment staffs are not only experiences, but also extremely supportive and will guide each travel nurse throughout their journey. They have highly efficient and customer-oriented support teams like Travel Relations and Housing and Credentialing Department that will ensure all the little details of the assignment is completely checked. Their team provides individual attention and focus to each RN.

Cirrus comprehensive medical plan under UMR/United Healthcare starts on Day 1 of employment. This medical plan provided to travel RNs is the same as their internal staffs (even their President!). They also offer a 401k with company match and a vesting period that is easy to complete. Sign-on Bonus, Referral Bonus and Loyalty Bonus are also provided. Their compensation package is customized to the needs of the travel RN and normally includes Per Diem, Housing Stipend or Corporate Housing, Travel Reimbursements, Licensure Reimbursements, and more! Payroll specialists are assigned to answer all of your questions. Don't forget to ask their Benefits Department about other optional employee-paid benefits such as vision and dental insurance, life insurance, supplemental insurance like cancer insurance, hospital stay insurance, and accidental insurance.

Cirrus is a privately owned company, with offices in Charlotte, NC and Fort Lauderdale, FL. Cirrus Medical Staffing has been in the Travel Nursing industry for over 13 years. Their longevity is indicative of their success in a very competitive healthcare field. In 2013, they were listed on Inc. Magazine's "5000 Fastest Growing Companies" in the US and are also recognized in SIA's 2015 Fastest Growing Staffing Companies.

For more information you can contact them at: 309 East Morehead Street, Suite 200 Charlotte, NC 28202. You can phone them at: 800-299-8132 or visit their website: *www.cirrusmedicalstaffing.com.*

~*~

Convergence Medical Staffing

Convergence Medical Staffing provides nationwide career opportunities for RN's, LPN's, OT's, PT's, COTA's, PTA's, MT's,

MLT's, Cath Lab Tech's, Surgical Techs, and a host of other allied health modalities.

They are medium sized company for a reason. Instead of placing volumes of nurses and other professionals all over the place, they keep their relationships personal. There are limitations on the number of travelers that their recruiters work with, ensuring dedication to the traveler's experience on each and every assignment. Each of their travelers have access to speak with the Managing Director at any time should they feel the need. They are open to constructive criticism and solve all issues TOGETHER with the traveler. No results are satisfying to anyone if both aren't involved in the resolution.

Convergence does have a clinical liaison that is available during business hours by email and phone. After hours, she is available by email. They are Joint Commission Certified. At this time, they do not belong to NATHO but plan on doing so very soon.

If there are recruiter/traveler issues, the Managing Director will have a conversation with the traveler and create the win/win. In some cases the traveler is reassigned to another recruiter. In other cases, a resolution is reached to create a better working relationship (this included counseling the recruiter and monitoring for compliance). In other instances, the Managing Director will work directly with the traveler to ensure traveler satisfaction.

Convergence provides Blue Cross/Blue Shield – Major medical and dental to their travelers. They do not offer vision insurance because there are no satisfactory vision plans that are worthwhile for the cost; however, they did replace vision with a $15,000 life insurance policy where the traveler appoints the beneficiaries of his/her choice. They do not offer a 401(k) at this time due to a lack of participation from their travelers.

Other benefits include: 24/7 emergency contact with a live person, paid medical benefits that effective day one of employment, weekly pay via direct deposit, travel pay to/from each assignment; license reimbursement, CEU reimbursement, and numerous bonus programs (for credentialing to loyalty to referrals). Starting shortly before the summer of 2016, each traveler will receive a AAA Travel Club membership, which entitles them to automobile services throughout the US and discounts for retail, restaurants, other goods/services throughout the US, city by city.

Convergence actually CARES that the traveler's experience is positive. They support their travelers when there are issues on their assignment (when reasonable...sometimes issues are about preferences, not issues). They have lasting relationships based on career guidance, mutual reliability and dependability, and they are honest in their dealings.

In Conclusion: All of their recruiters are experienced with travel healthcare professional placement. When they tell you something, you can take it to the bank. If they are wrong, they admit it and if a mistake were to occur related to your contract, they eat it. The traveler will always be in the drivers seat; however, they do require your full cooperation in order to get you what you want. That means they can be strict about you getting your required paperwork in order to get their travelers interviewed and for credentialing prior to a start date. It's necessary to treat both sets of information urgently in order to secure their travelers the best assignments.

For more information, contact them at: 5200 Seventy-Seven Center Drive, Suite 550, Charlotte, NC 28217. They can be phoned at: 980-207-5000 or visit their website: *cmstaff.com.*

~*~

Core Medical Staffing

Core Medical Group places RNs, LPNs, PTs, PTAs, OTs, OTAs, SLPs, CSTs, and Pharmacy Technicians nationwide.

They are a medium-sized, privately-owned company that has both the time and resources to give travelers full, personalized attention, and assist them with everything involved in the traveling process. This includes assisting the traveler with his/her application, housing, licensure assistance, and more.

Core Medical Group treats its nurses and allied health professionals like family members. Their recruiters consider it a common courtesy to give travelers their personal cell phone and home phone numbers, so that healthcare providers can reach their recruiters 24/7. They understand that their professionals work odd hours all across the country and they want them to know they can contact them any time for any reason. Core Medical recruiters are focused on and dedicated to the best interests of the traveler. They also cherish the relationships they build with their travelers and enjoy being part of their lives. They also have a clinical nurse liaison who is available 24/7.

They are Joint Commission Certified and recently passed a Joint Commission audit with no requirements for improvement identified. They are also a proud member of NATHO. All of their recruiters provide second-to-none customer service to their travelers. They develop deep friendships with their travelers and are with them through good times and bad, always with a sympathetic ear and with a drive to ensure their travelers' happiness. If there is ever an issue or if a traveler has concerns about his or her recruiter, Core Medical will reassign a traveler to another recruiter that will be a better fit.

Core Medical Group's insurance is provided by Anthem Blue Cross Blue Shield. They also offer Delta Dental Insurance and VSP Vision Insurance. All of these benefits are effective Day 1 of employment. They provide travelers with a Matching 401K and will match $0.50 to the dollar with at least a 1% contribution with a max match at a 6% contribution. Other benefits include: Club Core Med Annual Vacation Incentive where travelers can earn points for an annual trip to the Caribbean each year just for working with them; Weekly Pay With Direct Deposit; Referral Bonuses allowing travelers to earn cash or points toward their annual trip to the Caribbean; Travel Reimbursement; Licensure Assistance and Reimbursement; Tax Free Per Diem for lodging, meals, and incidentals (must be traveling away from permanent residence and qualify per the permanent tax residence form); Free Private Housing or Complete Relocation Assistance for those receiving lodging per diem; Free Unlimited Online CEUs through CE Direct; Free Medical Testing and Screening for any medical services required for a traveler's assignment; Free 50K Life Insurance; Healthcare Reimbursement Account (HRA); Veterinary Pet Insurance (VPI): Professional Liability: Workers Compensation: Employee Assistance Program: Short Term Disability (Voluntary): Additional Life and AD&D (Voluntary): Long Term Care Insurance (Voluntary); and a 529 College Savings Plan (Voluntary).

They don't lose contact with their travelers once they're on assignment. They are with them through every step of the process before, during, and after an assignment. Travelers can contact their recruiter 24/7 and also have a direct line to the Recruiting Manager 24/7. Core also offers industry-leading benefits, including an annual trip to the Caribbean for travelers who work with them. No other travel company offers this benefit. The trip is also an opportunity for their travelers and recruiters to meet and greet on an all-inclusive trip to the Caribbean. Lastly, they don't just place nurses and other traveling healthcare professionals, they build relationships and long-lasting friendships that they value and cherish.

For more information, you can contact them at: 2 Keewaydin Drive Salem, NH 03079, phone them at: 800-995-2673, or visit their website: *www.coremedicalgroup.com.*

~*~

Dzeel Clinical Healthcare Staffing

Dzeel Clinical Healthcare Staffing places Registered Nurses, Radiology Techs, Ultrasound Techs, RRT/CRT's, Cath Lab Tech's, Monitor Tech's Rehab – PT, OT, SLP, PTA, COTA.

They also provide Mental Health Workers (Sitters, Aides, and Advanced Practice Nurses) into nationwide travel contracts, local contracts, as well as, PRN, temp to perm, and direct hire positions.

Dzeel is a medium sized company who matches each HealthCare Professional (HCP), regardless of their discipline or specialty, to a single recruiter who is responsible for that HCP. As they work together, the recruiter and HCP build a relationship based on mutual respect and familiarity which fosters a sense of friendship. Friends are never numbers…friends are family. Dzeel does have a clinical nurse liaison that is available 24/7/365, and they are JCAHO certified.

To ensure that Dzeel HCP's are happy with their recruiters, leadership listens! If either gives the sense of dislike or discontent, leadership moves the HCP to another recruiter. If either openly asks, they move them no questions asked.

Dzeel offers all of their active HCP's health, vision and dental insurance through the national Blue Cross/Blue Shield network of providers. Every Dzeel HCP is automatically enrolled as a participant in Dzeel's Free Will Retirement Incentive program. For every hour a HCP works, Dzeel Clinical pays the HCP $.50 to apply towards the retirement option of the HCP's choice and Dzeel takes care of the taxes!

Other benefits include: CASH Referral Bonuses whether you work for them or not, Overtime and Holiday Pay in excess of 1.5, Travel Pay and Travel Lodging Pay, Education Reimbursements, Free Nationally Accepted CEU's to all HCP's, PTO per assignment, Sign On and Completion Bonuses, Parking Reimbursement, Company Provided Coverage for Workman's Comp and Liability and LIVE Personnel 24/7.

Dzeel in the Navajo language can be translated to mean "heartfelt strength," and that is exactly what you will find with them. They strive every day to serve their clients and staff with the ultimate in integrity and their demonstrated commitment to reliability. Dzeel Clinical was created to help meet the demands for high-quality healthcare professionals. Dzeel Clinical Healthcare (Clinical Staffing Inc.) is a woman owned HUB certified North Carolina based company. Dzeel Clinical is licensed by the State of North Carolina, Department of Health and Human Services, Division of Health Service Regulation to operate as a Nursing Pool Agency. As an established organization in North Carolina, their employee recruitment process is exceptional and their in-house procedures are proven. Dzeel is invested within their home state. In doing so they have become involved with the North Carolina Nurses Association, The North Carolina Psychiatric Association and they have been formally invited by the board and accepted as members of North Carolina Business Committee for Education which focuses on education and economic growth across North Carolina. Dzeel is also the only staffing company involved with Healthcare Works Partnership which is a regional organization addressing workforce needs in healthcare.

Their passion is building strong relationships while becoming the most reliable and educated Team in the health care industry. Their management philosophy is focused on three key words: Reliability, Relationships, and Education. They know that by focusing on these three words both internally and externally Dzeel is able to form the partnerships needed to provide the very best in patient care. Reliability for Dzeel Clinical is vital throughout their organization; from their internal team to their healthcare providers, being reliable is a critical piece of their partnership commitment. They employ professionals who are committed and dedicated in their specialty and also have a passion for patient care. Dzeel Clinical knows having a well-built relationship within an organization is essential to their success. What makes them unique among other supplemental staffing agencies is that they know each facility site is different and each manager will have their own procedures. Communication and making sure they follow the facility's requirements is priority number one for Dzeel Clinical. They connect their clients with appropriate Dzeel internal staff at the start of all relationships to ensure that communication flows smoothly 24/7 and any questions that arise can be answered quickly. In regards to their HCP's, Dzeel believes in open communication and encourages their HCP's to address any concerns or questions that may arise during their assignment. Their organization's emphasis on continuing education is one factor that clearly sets Dzeel Clinical Healthcare apart. They offer the practical and procedural courses to their healthcare providers in addition to giving attention to patient care within their training curriculum. Dzeel Clinical only submits skilled healthcare providers with an absolute minimum of one year of related experience to the assignment they are being presented for.

For more information contact them at 140 Commerce Parkway Suite 101, Garner, NC 27529. You can also phone them at 866-598-1523 or visit them on the web at: *www.dzeelclinical.com.*

~*~

Emerald Health Services

Emerald Health Services provide exciting travel, interim, and permanent opportunities for RNs across all nursing specialties. Their focus is on California; although, they do staff nurses nationwide. They are a small company that is rapidly growing.

Emerald has an experienced and dedicated team of recruiting professionals who pay close personal attention to the individual needs of every nurse. Emerald does have a clinical nurse liaison that is available 24/7. They are Joint Commission certified and belong to NATHO. Their Director of Recruiting works closely with their recruiters to ensure they are addressing the needs of each nurse. Their nurses are encouraged to speak with him directly if they ever feel they are not getting the excellent support and attention they deserve.

They offer a comprehensive suite of healthcare coverage, and they do provide a 401K plan to their nurses. Other benefits include a wide variety of generous travel incentives, allowances, and certification reimbursements.

They are a privately-owned company that builds their business on good word of mouth. Instead of spending money on marketing programs, they devote their resources to creating great compensation packages for their nurses and ensure that they generate a positive referral! They take great pride in their ability to help their nurses achieve their career goals. Give them a call and see how they can help you.

For more information, you can contact them at: 999 N Sepulveda, Suite 700 El Segundo, CA 90245. You can phone them at: 800-917-5055, or visit their website at: *www.emeraldhs.com.*

~*~

Expedient Medstaff

Expedient primarily staff RNs to beautiful locations throughout the 50 United States. They are a medium sized company that is operated by Registered Nurses. They understand nursing from a nurse's perspective. They assign a team to each one of their working nurses, which allows them to deliver exceptional service, quick answers, and guidance for their travelers.

Expedient is a Joint Commission Certified company that has two Clinical Nurse Liaisons and one is always available, every hour of every day, all year long.

Expedient Medstaff offers Blue Cross / Blue Shield which is available day-1. They also offer vision, dental, life, and short/long term disability. They also offer a 401k with a discretionary match. Other benefits they offer include: (1) Weekly pay with direct deposit and web access to pay records, (2) Travel to and from assignments, (3) Company provided housing or GSA schedule reimbursements, and (4) Customizable pay packages based on the needs of the RN.

Expedient is big enough to offer thousands of jobs and small enough to care about their travelers. As a smaller company Freedom gives more to their nurses, taking only 15–20% for overhead cost instead of the traditional 25–30% taken by most companies.

For more information, contact them at: One Heritage Place, Suite 250, Southgate, MI 48195. They can be reached by phone at: 877-367-8770, or visit them online at: *www.expedientmedstaff.com.*

~*~

Flexcare Medical Staffing

FlexCare Medical Staffing specializes in contracting RNs, and Allied Health who have at least one year of current experience, in acute care facilities throughout the nation.

FlexCare is the most well regarded travel nurse staffing company in the nation, and that's no accident. They abide by one simple philosophy: Travel Nursing Done Better. That's not just a fancy tagline—it really is the core of their business. Their program is built around you, which means highly-desired nationwide positions, top pay, and excellent service to ensure you have a great experience. FlexCare is the only staffing company that offers SinglePoint and MaxPay, two features that set them apart from everyone else.

No one enjoys being shuffled through multiple departments to make arrangements. It wastes time and raises annoyance levels. That's why with SinglePoint, you'll always have a single point of contact who takes care of all your assignment details and questions personally. No more runaround. No more repeating your information for the sixth time. Just one easy-to-reach person you can call for everything, from finding the ideal position to identifying housing options and managing compliance documentation. They stay right by your side with regular check-ins throughout your assignment, as well as perform weekly payroll audits to ensure your check is accurate before payday.

They're your new best friend, and like a true friend, they've got your back and make sure you're getting the maximum pay possible for every position, every time, no negotiation required—that's MaxPay. There's no need to negotiate, because they aren't holding anything back. Plus, unlike most staffing companies, they don't take a higher commission if the hospital's bill rate is increased. The higher the rate, the more money in your pocket, not theirs. At FlexCare, there is no hassle or stress when it comes to pay. They believe a good relationship starts with transparency and trust. With MaxPay, the goals are always aligned, and the focus is on finding you the perfect assignment with the pay you deserve.

With over 1300 client facilities in their nationwide network, FlexCare will not only find your ideal position, they will find it virtually anywhere you'd like to be. From coast to coast, they've built trusted relationships with hospital systems throughout the country and are able to offer their nurses the best of the best. Their recruiters go above and beyond to learn every region back to front so they can offer you thoughtful and informative insight into each possible position. Whether you'd prefer the fast-paced action of central Los Angeles, the laid back island lifestyle of Hawaii or the close-knit communities of the Midwest, they can make it happen for you. As a "preferred partner" for most of their hospitals, they provide exclusive access to premier job opportunities in the locations you want, and you're always offered MaxPay for the position.

The FlexCare team is comprised of some of the most dedicated and caring people on the planet. They began FlexCare as an alternative to the typical travel nursing experience; they wanted to create a company that nurses and hospitals could truly trust and depend on, much as your patients trust and depend on you. Clear, consistent, and honest communication are core principles of the service they provide. Don't take their word for it—the numbers speak for themselves. More than 94% of their workforce is comprised of nurses who continue to book new assignments through them, and 77% of new professionals come to them through referrals. They are a Joint Commission-certified provider for healthcare staffing services throughout the U.S., and they work tirelessly to support their clinicians and clients and make their lives easier so they can focus on what's really important.

For more information, you can contact them here: 990 Reserve Drive #250 Roseville, CA 95678. They call be reached by phone at: 866-564-3589, or visit their website at: *www.flexcarestaff.com.*

~*~

Freedom Healthcare

Freedom Healthcare has built its company offering opportunities and service to the RN community in all 50 states; however, they also offer opportunities in to the allied health community including physical rehab, radiology, and CSTs.

They are a medium sized company: large enough to offer hundreds of contracts but small enough to treat each traveler as an individual and have the ability to exercise flexibility that the largest companies do not.

Freedom Healthcare treats each nurse with respect as part of their company's mission statement, and all employees hired at Freedom are expected to demonstrate that value.

Their nurse manager is available during "business" hours; however, there is always a manager on call. They have been Joint Commission certified for over 10 years. Their organization does not belong to NATHO at this time.

The initial pairing of a nurse and recruiter is many times random. Most of the time, the pairing is a good match; however, in the event that the chemistry does not work, the nurse would make a request for a new recruiter. It is a simple process.

Freedom Healthcare has a comprehensive health insurance, including vision and dental that is offered through various national carriers. At this time they do not offer a 401K. In addition to Day-1 comprehensive health coverage, they offer assistance with nurse licensing, certification reimbursements on certain assignments, professional liability insurance, excellent housing options, as well as responsive customer service to their nurses.

Freedom Healthcare Staffing truly lives the core value that they treat each of their nurses with respect. Each member of the team gets to know their nurses and what their respective needs are. Although not every nurse has heard of their company, for each one that has, testimonials about Freedom's service always validate their claims.

Freedom healthcare is very proud to have built a company that prides itself on service to their nurses.

You can contact Freedom Healthcare Staffing at 3025 South Parker Road, Suite 800, Aurora, CO 80014. You also call them at: 866-463-0385 or visit their website: *www.freedomhcs.com.*

~*~

Fusion Medical Staffing

Fusion Medical Staffing places both nursing and allied healthcare travelers to include: RNs, LPNs, CNAs, CSTs, OTs, PTs, COTAs, PTAs, SLPs, and Lab staff nationwide.

They are a small privately owned company who makes personal service a top priority by having their structure set up to where a nurse has one point of contact which is their Nurse Recruiter. All of their employees also have their direct numbers to their cell phones to help with anything that may occur. They also have a nurse liaison that is available for employees during business hours.

Fusion Medical Staffing is Joint Commission Certified. They do not belong to NATHO yet, but are considering it. Their recruiters treat their nurses as number one by conducting extensive phone conversations and are willing to adjust things as necessary to make things work for all parties involved!

Their benefits include: Blue Cross Blue Shield for medical and Guardian for dental and vision, immediate contributions to a 401K with matching after one year of employment up to 5%. Their other benefits include: Top-notch customer service with a single point of contact, 401k that starts after 2,080 hours of service with a match or 100% of 3% and 50% of 2% through Hartford, Private Housing or Housing per diem, Weekly Per diem for meals, Referral Bonus of $500, Licensure Reimbursement, Travel Reimbursement, On Going Education Reimbursement, $300 a calendar year, Direct Deposit, and Vacation Hours with 40 hours received after 1,560 hours worked.

They are a smaller company for a reason and they don't want to become a larger company. They want to maintain their integrity and their commitment to keeping their travelers as their first priority! Only a smaller company can do that! They will grow by leaps and bounds in numbers, but they will never let the traveler feel like a number because of it!

The benefits of working with Fusion Medical: (1) You won't be just another number. You will be a valued employee, (2) They will be competitive with their pay packages, (3) You will receive top-notch customer service from your nurse recruiter, and (4) You will have a client manager that will be willing to put in the time to find you the job that you want.

To find out more about Fusion, you can find them at: 11808 Grant Street, Suite 100, Omaha, NE 68164. You can also reach them by phone at: 877-230-3885 or visit their website: *www.fusionmedstaff.com.*

~*~

Go Healthcare Staffing

Go Healthcare Staffing is a small company that has travel nursing assignments in all 50 states for travel nurse RNs. Their contracts vary in length of assignment but typically are 13 weeks or more, with opportunities for extensions. They are a full service company that is

Joint Commission Certified and has a clinical liaison 24 hours a day, 7 days a week.

All of their nurse recruiters have been in healthcare staffing for 10 years or more. They know the most important thing is ensuring a good fit between the travel nurse and the client. They strive to create long-term relationships with their travel nurses. They spend a significant amount of time speaking to their nurses about each opportunity to ensure it meets their needs and expectations.

Go Healthcare Staffing also offers excellent benefits packages including healthcare coverage from day 1 of employment and their compensation packages are some of the most competitive in the industry, so they deliver on their commitment to put nurses first. They're in it for the long haul and their collective experience has them focusing on the needs of their nurses.

They also have a "GO Happy" traveler program that contacts each nurse throughout their assignment to ensure they are happy, not only with the assignment, but also with their housing, their surroundings, etc. The GO Happy program is essentially a "concierge" service for their nurses to ensure they have what they need personally and professionally for a successful travel experience.

Go Healthcare Staffing recruiters take the time to get to know each traveler. Where possible, they even try to meet their travelers in person. If geography does not permit this, their recruiters make themselves available nights, weekends, or whenever convenient for the nurse to speak to them. They don't rush through their discussions, but instead take the time to fully understand the nurse and their professional and personal needs relative to their assignments. They make sure that the nurse fully understands their benefits packages, insurance coverage, and compensation packages to ensure they maximize what they have to offer.

All of their recruiters are veteran travel RN and healthcare recruiters so they all have experience in terms of the industry, what it takes to be successful and how important it is to treat nurses with respect given the incredibly important and demanding job that travel RNs have.

Go Healthcare Staffing's benefits are highlighted by health insurance with coverage from Day 1 of employment through United Healthcare. They also offer Vision and Dental insurance coverage as well and participation in the company 401(k) savings plan. Other benefits include: Weekly pay and competitive compensation; Direct deposit – Your paycheck is conveniently deposited into the bank account of your choice; Dedicated payroll support – payroll specialists are assigned to answer all of your questions; Medical coverage – healthcare coverage effective "day one" through United Healthcare; Prescription coverage; Dedicated 'Traveler Relations" contact designed to personally assist you during your assignment; 24 x 7 Emergency support coverage; Dental coverage – effective 30 days after first paycheck issued; Vision coverage – effective 30 days after first paycheck issued; Supplemental insurance options; Long-term disability; Life insurance; Professional liability insurance; Loyalty Bonus; Referral Bonus; Professional credentialing reimbursement; State licensure reimbursements; Travel reimbursements; and Private housing.

Go Healthcare Staffing is a new company, formed by experienced travel nursing recruiters and healthcare-related management that understand what travel nurses do, day in and day out. They understand the stress of the job, the ups and downs. They also understand there are many travel nurse staffing options out there for travel nurses. As a small company, they have put their resources into offering great benefits, very competitive compensation packages, and hiring great people to work with their nurses. They understand the frustration that travel RNs have with companies that "just don't get it" or recruiters that are in and out like revolving doors. They are committed, experienced, and know what it takes to create a lasting relationship with travel nurses. Give them a try and you'll see how they truly "put our money where our mouth is" and follow through with their commitments.

Go Healthcare Staffing is the place where nurses are put first every day! They will exceed your expectations and work for YOU!

You can find out more by contacting them at: 412 Louise Avenue Charlotte, NC 28204. Or you can phone them at 844-966-8773, or visit their website at: *www.gohealthcarestaffing.com.*

~*~

Healthcare Starz

Healthcare Starz places RNs, Allied Health, Radiology Techs, NPs, Pas, CRNAs, and Hospitalists all over the country, including Alaska, Hawaii, and the U.S. Virgin Islands. They are a small to medium sized company that is very family oriented. They treat all of their travelers as friends and like an extension of the family.

Although they are not Joint Commission Certified yet, they follow all Joint Commission policies and use their industry experience and long-term relationships to ensure they do things the “Right Way.” They have been working with travelers for over 15 years and many travelers still work with them because they treat them as if they were an extension of their own personal family. They become lifelong friends with all of their travelers. They always deliver on what they promise (No Bait and Switch) and always guarantee to call a traveler back on the same day if they leave them a message. Their clinical liaison is available at all hours of the day and night.

At Healthcare Starz they empower their recruiters to decide for themselves whether a nurse is a good fit for them. It’s part of their new hire training. They encourage their recruiters to work with travelers that have similar values and interests. As part of their training, they are taught to get to know the nurse or traveler first on a personal level and see if they get along and have good chemistry. They also train their recruiters to always put the nurse or traveler’s interests first before their own and teach them that if they approach everyone from the perspective of trying to help them, then they will build great long-term relationships.

Healthcare Starz offers Blue Cross National PPO and Dental and Vision Service through our nationwide Payroll Company. They also provide the best 401K in the industry with the most generous company match. They match a traveler’s contributions dollar for dollar up to the first 3% of their contribution and 50% on the next 2% of their contribution. So, if a traveler just puts in 5% of their pay, they will match them 4% which gives them an 80% return on their money not even factoring in any investment return gains. The Best Part: The traveler is 100% vested in their match immediately! There is no 5 or 6 year vesting schedule like most all of the other companies out there. They believe that their phenomenal match and immediate vesting is a great recruiting tool for travelers who want to build up their retirement dollars quickly and/or those who have not started but want to make catch up contributions, taking advantage of the great match they offer. Healthcare Starz not only reimburses for licensure, certifications, but they also provide an EAP “Employee Assistance Program” for nurses/

travelers. This program is 100% confidential and allows travelers to talk with a counselor if they need to discuss any personal matters that may be affecting their lives.

What makes Healthcare Starz different is that every traveler has access to the owner of the company, Monte Kasten, if they have an issue they need resolved. They don't have to talk to someone, who then has to talk with someone else, before a decision gets made. They believe in having a single point of contact for each nurse, which is their recruiter and that recruiter becomes the lifeline for the traveler. If anything ever needs to get escalated, there are not multiple layers of management to go through to get things resolved.

When you have your first conversation with a recruiter, you will immediately recognize the difference and positive vibe you get when they focus on what's most important to you, not them. By always doing what is in the best interest of their travelers, they have been able to build lifelong relationships with all of their travelers. They would be very honored to have you join the Healthcare Starz family of travelers who are treated with honor, respect, and appreciation.

Healthcare Starz caters to newbies! If you're a First Time Traveler, they excel at making you feel comfortable through the whole process and they coach you on how to navigate the benefits and challenges you'll have by becoming a traveler. They would be very honored to talk with you and invite you to give them a call.

For more information, contact them at: 5717 South Dixie Highway, Suite #334, Miami, FL 33167. You can phone them at 888-777-4920 or visit them on the web at: *www.healthcarestarz.com.*

~*~

Health Providers Choice

Health Providers Choice is a mid-sized private owned company held corporation, which offers RNs, LPNs, CNAs, OTs, PTs, STs, RTs, and CSTs throughout the United States and Canada.

All nurses working with Health Providers Choice are employees of Health Providers Choice (W-2). They are able to offer assignment terms of 4 weeks up to 26 weeks in length for travel and local RN's and flexible scheduling for casual/per-diem RN's. Health Providers Choice specializes in nurse placement however they also place certified scrub techs and a few allied health personnel. You can visit their website for a complete list of their current positions. They place all specialties, and have a national client base. They are able to offer assignment terms of 4 weeks up to 26 weeks in length for travel and local healthcare providers and flexible scheduling for casual/per-diem healthcare providers. HPC was nurse founded in 2001 and remains nurse owned and operated.

They pride themselves on living their mission and their values. They honor each person in their organization and because of their commitment there are no numbers, everyone is a very important professional in their organization. They take time to build mutually beneficial relationships with the nurses they partner with as well as their clients. As a nurse owned and operated organization, the value of their nurses is inherent in the HPC Culture. Health Providers Choice understands and appreciates the challenges and rewards of providing patient care and they strive to help with the challenge and consistently find ways to help make it as rewarding as possible. From the introduction of their organization throughout your employment you will receive a personal and high touch experience. It is through the relationships their recruiters have with the employees they serve that earned Health Providers Choice bragging rights in the travel nurse industry. Greater than 65% of all nurses working with Health Providers Choice refer at least one colleague.

During every phase of the employment process including credentials, placement, housing, travel, and professional advocacy, HPC is available 24 hours, 7 days a week, and 364 days a year. Health Providers Choice has a 24-hour on-call as well as a Chief Nursing Officer available around the clock for clinical issues that may arise and nurse/patient advocacy. Health Providers Choice has been Joint Commission Certified since 2005 and is a founding member of NATHO.

Health Providers Choice takes great care in the selection process of their recruitment team. All of their recruiters have long tenures in the healthcare industry working either as a nurse, an allied professional, or healthcare recruiter. They are well educated in the industry and the roles they are recruiting for which allows for great synergy early in the process. Also, all of HPC's recruiters are a testament to the corporate mission and value structure, which allows for a mutually respectful partnership between themselves and the nurses they serve. Strong relationships are essential for their success. Health Providers Choice highlights their recruitment team on their website and each recruiter has a personal information page to allow nurses to review the team and find the best fit. Nurses working for Health Providers Choice can choose to change recruiters at anytime if they wish to experience a new relationship within their company.

Health Providers Choice has Blue Cross Blue Shield Medical/ Dental/Vision. They offer 4 low deductible, Cobra qualified plans, with first day coverage to choose from. They also offer 401K through Lincoln Financial. They have a profit sharing match plan after the participant is vested. (ERISA Plan)

Other benefits include: Short-Term Disability Plan-13 weeks; Voluntary Long Term Disability; Life Insurance of 50K; Death and Dismemberment Insurance of 50K; Unlimited Free CEU's; Reimbursement for BLS/ACLS; Paid Pre-hire and yearly medical physicals and titers; Licensure Reimbursement; Employee Assistance Program through BCBS; Furnished Housing for Traveler; Tax Benefit Plan (Federal Tax Per-diem) for qualified travelers; Vacation Accrual and Sick Pay Accrual Available; Awards, Completion Bonus's, Sign on Bonus's are available on some of the assignments; and a very competitive referral bonus plan

Health Providers Choice is nurse owned and operated. All decisions that are made within the company are made by nurses for nurses. The nurse founders of HPC are dedicated to the success of their colleagues. HPC uses full disclosure and open negotiation allowing for mutual decision making and collaborative contracting. They are proud to have high retention rates and employee satisfaction scores that are 68% higher than the national average.

At Health Provider Choice their mission is to exceed the service and quality expectations of their customers, the community, the professionals they employ, and themselves. They are true to this mission and are always excited to have another industry professional join them in successfully executing it.

You can contact them at: 715 E. South Blvd. Suite 100A Rochester Hills, Michigan 4830. They can be phoned at: 888-299-9800, or visit their website at: *www.hpcnursing.com.*

~*~

Host Healthcare

Host Healthcare offers positions for all types of RNs, as well as therapy positions for PTs, OTs, SLPs, PTAs, and COTAs in all 50 states.

They are a medium size private company. Their goal is to offer all the jobs and benefits of a large company while offering the service and attentiveness of a smaller company.

Host Healthcare cannot overstate how much they value their nurses and the services they provide to their patients. They care about each nurse as an individual. Their goal is not only to find their nurses the best assignment, but also to act as their career counselor and friend.

They are a Joint Commission certified staffing company who has a full-time Clinical Nurse Liaison who is on call 24 hours per day.

Host Healthcare recruiters have recruitment managers who periodically check in with each nurse while they are on assignment. If a nurse does not feel that his or her recruiter is a good fit, the recruitment manager will assign a different recruiter to the nurse based on what the nurse is looking for in a recruiter.

They offer day one medical insurance. It is a PPO insurance plan through Aetna Healthcare. The plan covers all medical emergencies as well as doctors' visits, specialist visits, special procedures, etc. We also offer vision and dental insurance plans for their nurses. They also offer a 401(k) plan for their nurses through Principal Financial Group with match 50% of the nurse's contributions.

Host Healthcare also offers deluxe corporate housing or a tax-free housing allowance, sign-on and completion bonuses for certain assignments, paid travel expenses, free CEUs, tuition reimbursement for recent graduates, 24-hour support, and a dedicated "nurse concierge" to help you make the most of your assignment.

Their people make the difference. They only hire the best nurse recruiters and support staff. Their goal is not only to match their nurses with the best assignments but also to make a difference in the lives of their nurses by providing them with exceptional service and support. Their nurses can be confident that they are working with experienced travel nursing professionals who deeply care about them as individuals.

Host Healthcare is dedicated to going "above and beyond" to make each assignment memorable. A few key examples include: providing travelers with rental cars, assisted with arranging activities for their nurses in their area, and personally taking their nurses out for dinner and drinks if they are visiting their area or if they are visiting beautiful San Diego!

In addition, they believe in compensating their nurses generously for the work that they do. Their nurses make on average 5–10% more in take home pay compared to other companies. Combined with the other benefits that they offer, they believe that they have the best all-around package for their nurses.

To find out more, you can contact them at: 540 Towne Centre Drive, Suite 150 San Diego, CA 92101. You can also phone them at: (800) 585-1299, or visit their website at: *www.hosthealthcare.com.*

~*~

IPI Travel

IPI Travel specializes in RN's, OTs, PTs, STs, and Nurse Practitioners. They have nationwide assignments.

IPI is a privately owned and operated mid-western company located in Noblesville, IN. They treat each traveler as a unique individual by customizing each travel assignment and asking the question, "What are you looking for in an assignment?" Travel staff is always available to answer questions, with a common of each IPI travel staff member to make travelers feel welcome and valued from the first hello.

A call representative is available 24/7/365 and will return emergency pages within 30 minutes. They realize that IPI is a lifeline while on assignment and they are ready to help in any way possible. A clinical nurse liaison is also available as needed.

IPI is Joint Commission Certified with 100% compliance with all re-certifications thanks to their wonderful staff and travelers!

IPI's policy requires their team members to work together to meet the needs of the travelers. If the traveler isn't clicking with the staffing specialist, simply request another staffing specialist. Senior management is committed to finding the right fit for everyone.

Medical insurance coverage is provided by Cigna, Dental and Vision and is at no additional cost to the travelers. IPI also offers a generous 401k program with company match and only a 3-year vesting schedule.

Other benefits include: paid vacation, travel pay, bonuses, as well as an allocation for "life happens" with missed shifts during an assignment. But it's the little things that really differentiated IPI from everyone else. From personal service, extras during the assignment, saying thanks and doing things when it's least expected, those little things still mean something. Travelers can now enjoy IPI's weekly per diem pay.

From the president: On many occasions I have been asked the question, "Why should I choose IPI Travel?" I don't have to think twice when I answer this question; IPI is a direct reflection of many years of hard work and dedication. We treat each traveler as a unique individual. Customizing each travel assignment, asking the question, "What are you looking for in a partner, what are you looking for in an assignment?" These are the principles IPI Travel has maintained since 1999. To this day we demand continued excellence from all of IPI's internal staff as well as their travelers. Our goal is for each of their customers to have a feeling of "Wow" when interacting with the IPI team. IPI achieves the "Wow" factor with each placement by on-time delivery of completely detailed contracts, special thanks before and during the assignment, detailed housing packages, free CE's, and a knowledgeable staff to help with all traveling details! We believe in holding staff and travelers accountable and I expect wonderful things from all of them. IPI wouldn't be successful without their great travel professionals, account managers, staffing specialist, and support staff. In addition to all the services IPI offers we also continue to develop client relationships throughout the United States, giving their travelers a huge network of resources and the flexibility for unlimited travel assignment choices. Each assignment is custom-designed around the traveler. IPI Travel understands healthcare professionals are in great demand; this is why we are committed to making your travel assignment rewarding and hassle-free. I will personally guarantee your assignment will be everything we promised. For questions regarding IPI Travel or comments please feel free to call."

IPI values their travelers, and, they work every day to improve their processes and service. Just doing isn't good enough, being the best is what they strive for.

For more information you can contact them at: 14701 Cumberland Road, Suite 140 Noblesville, IN 46060. You can phone them at: 800-322-9796, or visit their website: *www.ipitravel.com.*

~*~

Jackson Nursing Professionals

Jackson Nurse Professionals is a large RN staffing firm that has nationwide contracts. They are a Joint Commission Certified Company as well as a member of NATHO. Nurses are the lifeblood of their company, so their recruiting method is completely relationship focused.

Their team lets the nurse take the lead, putting their needs and goals ahead of their own preferences or opinions while always being available for expert guidance and counsel. To assure that nurses never feel like a number, they implemented several "check-in" points during the on-boarding process and throughout the contract to continually foster an open dialogue with Jackson Nurses and to handle any last-minute needs, issues, or situations that arise as quickly as possible.

Jackson Nurse recruitment managers do a personal follow-up with nurses to make sure they're benefiting from the relationship they have with their current recruiter. If the nurse or recruiter feels they aren't a match, their recruitment managers reassign the nurse to a recruiter that more closely aligns with their personality or preferences.

Their benefits include: Blue Cross Blue Shield medical insurance with elective benefits through Guardian, a company match 401k investment option, CEU and License Reimbursement, Loyalty Bonuses, Life Insurance, Short-Term Disability, Long-Term Disability, Housing and Relocation Costs (within IRS regulations), Referral Rewards income, and Referral Bonuses.

Jackson Nurse Professional's commitment to nurses goes beyond their travel contract; their hope is that they get a chance to make an impact in their communities through their various Giving Back campaigns. As a member of Jackson Healthcare's family of staffing companies, they were founded on one principle: to improve the lives of patients, families, and their communities.

Jackson not only serves health systems and providers nationwide, but they champion local, national, and international charitable work.

For more information, they can be contacted at: 3452 Lake Lynda Dr., Suite 200, Orlando, FL 32817. They also can be phoned at: 888-300-5132, or visit their website at: *www.jacksonnursing.com.*

~*~

Medical Solutions

Medical Solutions offer opportunities for RNs ranging from staff RN to RN management. They offer jobs for LPN, OT, ST, and PT.

Their jobs are located all over the 50 states. They are the third largest travel nurse staffing company in the nation. They have approximately 200 full-time internal employees between their four locations in Omaha, San Diego, Cincinnati, and Tupelo. They are currently privately held.

Their company culture is all about treating people well and celebrating their individual talents and successes. This spirit extends through their Career Consultants (their name for "Recruiters") to their Travelers, who they also consider a part of their team. Ultimately this positive attitude extends into the hospital, which makes for great patient care and happy nurses. They don't just staff nurses; they help them build their careers. But they also care deeply for them as individuals. Their Career Consultants work to be both professional and personal with their Travelers, and their work is not done when a nurse is placed. Their Career Consultants check in to make sure all is going well and are there throughout an assignment to provide any support a Traveler may need. And because they have such extraordinary Travelers, they also love to tell their stories on their blog.

At this time, Medical Solutions has four internal RNs who act as Clinical Nurse Liaisons. They have a 24-hour on call emergency line which can easily connect to one of them 24 hours a day, 7 days a week. Quality assurance is also provided through being Joint Commission certified and a NATHO member. Medical Solutions was one of the first Joint Commission certified companies, and their President, Craig Meier, sits on the NATHO board.

Initially, their Career Consultants spend a lot of time getting to know the person up front during the qualifying process. They ask a lot of questions to make sure it is going to be a good match personality-wise as well as a fit for what the Traveler is looking for in a company. They also have managers who call their Travelers within the first 1–2 weeks of their assignments to check in and ask for feedback on how the recruiter is doing, and they do the NPS surveys to gauge customer satisfaction and identify any areas of improvement. Overall, they work hard to encourage an open forum so that travelers feel comfortable addressing any concerns they have with Career Consultants, but if they are still not entirely comfortable addressing the issues directly with their Career Consultant, they will always have other means to do so.

Medical Solutions offers day one United Healthcare coverage, and in 2013 they drastically lowered insurance costs for their Travelers! With a larger contribution from Medical Solutions, they now offer basic, single policy medical plans starting at just $15 per week. They offer day one dental benefits through Guardian. For vision they offer Vision Access or Vision VSP. Vision Access benefits come free with paid dental plan enrollment.

The benefits with Medical Solutions are never-ending! They are a pet-friendly company and they offer loyalty and referral bonuses, 24-hour customer care, an RN to BSN program, license and certificate reimbursement, their Go Rewards program, which gives Travelers access to all kinds of discounts on phone service, scrubs, rental cars, pet supplies, and more. They offer great paid private housing.

They also award one Traveler of the Month and one Rising Star of the Month (the latter a first-time Traveler with them) in order to reward their Travelers for excellent service based upon hospital evaluations. They sponsor a lot of really cool contests with great prizes throughout the year! They also offer day one 401k through Nationwide. They offer a traditional 401k as well as a Roth plan. Company match is 50% of the first 3% elected.

Their amazing people and quality of customer service is really what sets them apart. They came up with nine core values that they live and work by, which really explain what's important to them and what sets them apart. They are: (1) Remain flexible and embrace change. (2) Show passion for work and have fun doing it. (3) Challenge yourself and strive for excellence. (4) Create a positive experience with everyone you encounter. (5) Treat people like you want to be treated. (6) Be an expert at your job. (7) Be proactive not reactive. (8) Focus on the solution, not the problem. (9) Use open and honest communication to build trust.

More interesting facts about Medical Solutions! (1) They have a lot of fun online. Check out their Facebook page, and the Medical Solutions blog on their site. (2) They think Travel Nurses are so special that in 2013 they created and celebrated the first-ever Travel Nurses Day, October 11, 2013. (3) Give them a call! If you like fun people and an agency that focuses on its Travelers' satisfaction and not the numbers, then traveling with Medical Solutions is for you.

For more information, you can contact them at: 1010 North 102nd

Street, Suite 300 Omaha, NE 68114. They can be phoned at: 866-633-3548, or visit them at their website: *www.medicalsolutions.com.*

~*~

Medical Staffing Solutions, INC

Medical Staffing Solutions, Inc. is a certified by the Joint Commission Certified company that specializes in providing temporary and supplemental placement of healthcare professionals, including nurses and allied healthcare professionals throughout the US.

They are a medium sized company who doesn't outsource anything! All recruiting, credentialing, and payroll is done by their employees in their office. They are big enough to serve their employees, but small enough to take care of their employees on a personal basis. Their recruiters work not only as a recruiter, but as a career coach as well. They ask questions and listen to their nurses needs to determine the best fit for their nurses and therapists.

Medical Staffing Solutions, Inc. offers competitive salaries, private and furnished housing, traveler-friendly facilities, and first day benefits! Also available are life insurance and 401k options. Becoming a travel nurse is an exciting career! Choose Medical Staffing Solutions, Inc. to represent you when it comes to your assignments.

Most agencies advertise that they are the best or largest or something similar to that. At MSSI, they understand that it truly is a partnership between the agency and the employees, so they do everything that is in their control to grow that partnership resulting in both the agency and the employee being very satisfied. They don't advertise that they are the biggest or best. They are all about providing the traveling nurse or traveling therapist an opportunity to work with an agency that they can truly rely on to be honest and hardworking on their behalf. They also maintain a dedicated support staff available to you 24/7.

For more information, contact them at: 1805 Kern Avenue, Rice Lake, Wisconsin 54868. The can be reached by phone at: 877-217-9825, or find them on the web at: *www.travelmssi.com.*

~*~

Medical Staffing Solutions, LLC

Medical Staffing Solutions, LLC offers career opportunities in all nursing including RN, LPN and CNA, all therapies, and all allied health. They staff every medical profession, other than physicians. They are a medium sized company that is not only nurse owned and operated but a National Women Owned Business Enterprise. Their assignments are located nationwide, and they specialize in Alaska and Hawaii. In fact, they are one of the number one providers for Hawaii.

They are Joint Commission certified and belong to NATHO. To assist you with any clinical needs they have a nurse on call 24/7 that can help. They also do a clinical interview on every nurse before they take an assignment.

Medical Staffing Solutions, LLC, specializes in making a great fit between Traveler and Recruiter. They work with the specialty and location. If a traveler does request a certain recruiter or needs to change related to a conflict, they absolutely honor that request. They want their travelers to be happy and know that they are not alone.

They have day one insurance that is provided by Blue Cross/Blue Shield. Vision, dental, and life insurance is also provided for their travelers. After working for them for 90 days, they match 4% of the healthcare provider's contribution.

Being a nurse owned company, they have been where you are. They pride themselves in making each package individualized based on the healthcare provider's needs. They want every assignment to be a great experience, and they will go the extra mile to make sure that happens.

When we asked CEO, Melanie Theriac, RN, about what makes them stand out she stated, "Our Mission at Medical Staffing Solutions, LLC is: Patient's First. Our philosophy in decision making is doing what is best for the patient and the rest will fall in place. Our motto: "Healthcare with purpose." Becoming a travel healthcare professional is a choice and we want you to know that we will treat you as we would want to be treated."

For more information, you can contact them at 601 N Kentucky Ave. Suite A, Evansville, IN 47725. You can phone them at 812-469-6877 or visit their website at: *www.mssmedicalstaffing.com.*

~*~

Nationwide Nurses

Nationwide Nurses has career opportunities include short and long term travel assignments for Nurses, Allied, and Tech's.

Their career opportunities include short and long term travel assignments for Nurses, Allied, and Tech's. They are experienced and committed to build lasting relationships with their Nursing Partners. Their recruiters are available 24/7 to assist you with any situation during the course of your employment/assignment and offer personalized service to each and every Partner.

Nationwide Nurses offers a health benefit package tailored to meet your individual needs. Nationwide provides competitive financial support, regardless of the duration of your travel assignment. They also provide you a dedicated representative to assist you in customizing a health plan for you individually or for your family. Your benefits continue without interruption, as long as there is no more than a 30 day break in assignment annually.

Nationwide Nurses strives to get their nurses the best pay package! Highest hourly wages available, free private housing or a generous stipend, weekly pay through direct deposit, lucrative completion bonuses along with referral and loyalty bonuses. Other benefits include: travel pay up front, rental car stipends, overtime opportunities, personal crisis assistance, licenses paid in full, health insurance stipends, along with other great incentives and perks.

The personalized service that their nurses receive and peace of mind is what makes their company different than all the rest. Their recruiters truly go above and beyond to ensure that things go off without a hitch. In the event that something doesn't go as planned; your personal recruiter is available to you 24/7 to help get things back on track. Most of their travelers have been with us for years! They continue to travel with Nationwide because of how well they are respected and treated!

For more information, you can find them here: 9435 E. 51st Street, Suite A, Tulsa, OK 74145. They can be phoned at: 866-836-8773, or visit them online here: *www.nationwidenurses.com.*

~*~

OneStaff Medical

OneStaff Medical is a nationwide healthcare staffing firm focusing on the placement of Nursing, Allied, and Rehab Therapy Professionals. Make OneStaff Medical your, "One Solution for Staffing."

OneStaff Medical is a privately owned company based in Omaha, NE. What is their philosophy? Simply put, their philosophy is, "We believe in respect, honesty, dedication, hard work and professional courtesy. We understand communication is important to both their employees and their partner healthcare facilities."

Each healthcare professional has a dedicated recruiter in which handles all aspects of the assignment – 24/7. OneStaff Medical also has a dedicated Nurse Liaison that is available during and after normal business hours.

OneStaff Medical is Joint Commission Certified and has been since 2011. They also belong to various healthcare organizations: American Staffing Association, Staffing Industry Analyst, AWHONN, ENA, AORN, and AHRA. Their belief in these partnerships, knowledge is power for their people.

Benefits include: Cigna medical insurance, MetLife dental (both of which offer two plan options), VSP vision, Slavik 401k, Group Life and AD&D (company paid to $10,000) with additional amounts available to purchase, Short Term Disability and Critical Illness Insurance all offered through The Standard.

Other benefit offerings include, private housing or weekly housing allowance, weekly Per Diem, travel reimbursement, referral bonus of $500, license reimbursement and weekly direct deposit with online access to deposit records. OneStaff also offers to their staff corporate discounts through Extended Stay America and National/Enterprise car rental.

The company culture is that everyone is part of the OneStaff family – and that includes their travel staff. Per staff member's words to describe the company, "Family, Growth, Driven, Teamwork and Fun." Using these key words to conduct their everyday business, allows them to provide the highest quality service and experience travelers want and need.

Evidence of the company's success: 2x recipient of the Top Ten Travel Companies by Highway Hypodermics, 2015 Inc. 500, 2015 and 2106 Best Staffing Firms to Work for – Staffing Industry Analyst, Inavero 2016 Best of Staffing for Client's and Talent Award and 2016's Best Places to Work in Omaha.

OneStaff Medical's commitment to its internal and external staff is that no matter how fast or large they grow; everyone will be treated as an integral part of the OneStaff family!

For more information, you can check them out at: 11819 Miracle Hills Dr, Suite 101, Omaha, NE 68154. You can also phone them at: 877-783-1483, or visit their website at: *www.onestaffmedical.com.*

~*~

PPR Travel Nursing

PPR is a medium sized company that places RNs nationwide. As the name of the company implies, PPR Travel Nursing is dedicated and specialized in one thing…travel nursing.

PPR is known in the industry for their unique culture, best in industry customer service and their brand promise, "We Put You First".

For over 20 years, Recruiters, Client Account Managers, Human Resources and other support departments such as Payroll, Housing and Quality Management all pride themselves on creating the best employment experience for their travelers.

PPR offers nationwide assignments, competitive salaries, excellent Day 1 benefits and the best referral bonus in the industry—$1000.

In addition to all the support you will receive along the way, PPR also has multiple clinicians on staff available for help, advice, and guidance on any issues you might face while on assignment.

PPR's focus around customer service will build your trust, comfort, knowledge, and confidence in both the industry and your individual experience.

For more information you can visit them at: 333 First Street North, Suite 200, Jacksonville Beach, FL 32250. They can be reached by phone here: 866-581-5038, or you can visit their website at: *www.pprtravelnursing.com.*

~*~

PRCS Healthcare

PRCS is a mid-sized staffing firm, which equates to more competitive pay packages for their travelers. They offer RN, RT, and rehab assignments nationally.

Being a mid-size firm owned and operated by previous healthcare travelers, PRCS prides itself in caring for and knowing their travelers. Many of their travelers have been with them for years, some near a decade. Their travelers are a direct reflection of their firm and its quality. Their phones are answered 24/7, and they have a clinical liaison that is available. They have been a Joint Commission certified company since May 2010.

Nurses are paired with a nurse recruiter dedicated to their clinical specialty. They also account for gender and personality preferences when assigning recruiters.

PRCS has outstanding United health, dental and vision benefit packages offered to travelers, with custom package options. Other benefits include: 401k, referral bonuses, licensing reimbursement, certification reimbursements, and round-trip travel reimbursement.

What makes PRCS different? (1) They have been in business since 1981 (long standing), (2) They are Joint Commission certified with quality standards, (3) PRCS is owned and operated by previous healthcare clinicians which familiar with clinical settings and travel staffing. They understand the environment nurses work in, and the challenges they face caring for patients in a high stress environment, (4) They are a mid-size firm and can offer the most competitive pay packages, (5) PRCS knows and cares for their travelers. As a result, their business has been established largely by referrals from happy employees.

Their motto at PRCS is "Work hard, Play Hard." They are committed to working hard for their travelers and playing hard to have some fun with them!

For more information, you can contact them at: 4835 E. Cactus Rd #240, Scottsdale AZ 85254. They can also be phoned at: 888-508-2111, or visit them on the web at: *www.prcshealthcare.com.*

~*~

Premier Healthcare Professionals

Premier Healthcare Professionals (PHP) offers nationwide assignments for RN's, LPN's, OT's, ST's, and PT's throughout the 50 States. PHP and its subsidiary Bridge Staffing, can also offer International assignments (when available) through their company owned offices in England, Australia, and South Africa. It is now privately owned by its management team and should be classified as a medium-sized business.

The level of care and support provided to their Healthcare Professionals is PHP's major focus. Most of their staff have worked for the company for over 12 years and they believe that they have built up a vast experience on how their Healthcare Professionals should expect to be treated. They are continually amazed by the 'horror' stories they hear about from professionals wanting to switch from other staffing companies. Each of the PHP Professionals is assigned to a personal recruiter who is tasked with understanding their professionals' needs and identifying the most suitable assignments. The recruiters are continually assessed for how many professionals continue to re-contract with them at the end of each assignment.

PHP is Joint Commission Certified and a member of NATHO. As a company they strive to provide the best possible service to their clients and professionals alike. Certification by the Joint Commission and membership of NATHO is an integral part of this process. They also have a full-time RN on staff that has responsibility for being a Clinical Nurse Liaison. She is available 24/7.

PHP understands that its Healthcare Professionals are human and each have personal targets and personalities. The recruiters are trained to both recognize and adapt to the fact that each of their clinical colleagues are different and have varying requirements. Management makes itself readily available to all Healthcare Professionals should any issues arise. They work quickly to resolve any such matters and always make the requirements of their Healthcare Professionals their main priority.

PHP is recognized for its industry leading pay and benefits packages. Apart from providing first day, free health coverage with BCBS, it also provides dental, life, long and short term disability if required. Their comprehensive benefits package includes the option of a company match 401k plan if required. In addition to the insurance options above, they also offer free housing, housing allowance, contribution to utilities, sign-on bonuses, relocation, referral bonuses, CEU, and many, many more financial incentives. There is of course also the benefit of working for one of the longest serving and most awarded staffing companies in the world!

PHP truly is special. Many of its Healthcare Professionals continue to trust in the company and have completed multiple assignments over several years. The facts are that they know what they are doing…they have been doing the same thing for 25 years. Their staff are some of the most experienced in the industry. On average each of them has been employed by PHP for over 12 years. They place in all 50 States in the USA and internationally. On top of all of this they have won numerous awards within the industry for their pay and service standards. Not many staffing companies can boast all of this.

Apart from all of the outstanding service standards that you can expect, PHP will never be beaten on a genuine pay or benefits package. They recognize that healthcare professionals have a choice when it comes to staffing companies. They simply have to offer the best packages in order to grow and flourish.

For more information, you can contact them here: 3275 Market Place Boulevard, Suite 275, Cumming, Georgia 30041. They can be reached by phone at: 866-296-3247, or visit their website at: *www.travelphp.com.*

~*~

Primetime Healthcare

Prime Time Healthcare has CNA, LPN, and RN travel contracts in all 50 states and are exploring international contracting business. They are staffing in Hospitals, Nursing Homes, Clinics, Corrections, and any other environments that will accept their contracted services.

Prime Time Healthcare consistently follows up weekly, and you also are provided with the recruiter's cell phone number. Prime Time Healthcare and their recruiters will send gifts throughout the year to nurses to show their constant appreciation. They also send appraisals to the nurse to find out how they are doing. Prime Time Healthcare Management will send out appraisals on the recruiter to the nurse. Also management occasionally calls to ensure everything is going good. They also have a clinical liaison nurse who is on call 24 hours a day.

Prime Time Healthcare has started the process becoming Joint Commission certified which should be issued in 2016.

Prime Time Healthcare offers insurance for health, dental, and vision. Other benefits include 401k, per diem rates, rental cars, flights, shuttles, weekly direct deposit, flexible housing and amenities, reimbursement for licensing/certifications, and immunizations.

Prime Time Healthcare is a leader in travel nursing setting themselves apart with their industry knowledge, competitive and flexible pay rates, referral bonuses for ALL travelers, and additional bonuses for contests during the year along with special gifts for holidays and healthcare appreciation weeks throughout the year. They will continue to match or beat any pay package out there at the same facility.

For more information, you can visit them at: 14811 Shepard Street, Omaha, NE. 68138. They can also be contacted by phone at: 402-933-6700, or visit their website at: *www.primetimehealthcare.com.*

~*~

Randstad Healthcare

Randstad currently places RNs, LPNs, CSTs, Advanced Practice Professionals, Case managers, and Allied Health Professionals – including NPs, Pas, Certified Midwife's, Certified Nurse Specialists, and CRNA. They also staff Cath Lab Technicians, Medical Assistants, Pharmacists, Pharmacy Techs, Phlebotomists, and Ultrasound/ Sonographers.

Randstad Healthcare places candidates in Travel/Locum Tenens, Short-Term Contracts, and Permanent positions which are nationwide. They are a Joint Commission certified company along with a being a founding and current member of NATHO.

Randstad Healthcare is a part of Randstad, the second largest staffing company in the world. They are a publically traded on the NYSE. Randstad works hard to know their candidates. They work hard to know their clients. It is through their work ethic that they are able to create the best connections that have the most impact at America's top healthcare facilities. It is professionals coupled with expert recruiters that give nurses the inside track to drive the nurses' career. With over 25 years of experience, their industry knowledge takes you to where you want to be in the healthcare profession.

Throughout Randstad Healthcare, you will find that they bring an unparalleled passion to the way they work together. They focus on customer service and personalized attention with both their professionals and clients. Their dedicated team wants to get to know you, and ensure success through your entire career at Randstad! They openly welcome feedback and strive to make the best job matches to set you up for success.

Melissa Knybel, RN, BSN, is the Clinical Nurse Liaison and Vice President of Clinical Services, Compliance and Quality Management. Melissa is available 24 hours a day, 7 days a week via the emergency line or email. Melissa has over 10 years of clinical experience, and genuinely understands how important it is to have a resource to seek advice, or in some cases, act as an advocate.

Randstad Healthcare understands just how important it is to have a solid recruiter-nurse relationship to ensure a positive traveler experience. Many of their recruiters have a focus on a specific nursing specialty to ensure optimal match between the candidate, the recruiter, and the assignment. They rely on their candidates to keep an open, honest line of communication, so that they can be aware when things are going well, or if something requires a change or further attention. They frequently survey their candidates to ensure that the appropriate level of service is being delivered in all areas.

Randstad offers every travel and contract employee a choice of CIGNA medical plans, a dental plan, and a vision plan. Candidates are eligible for the Randstad 401K retirement plan, with company match.

Aside from medical related benefits and 401K enrollment option, Randstad Healthcare are offers travelers: Free, private, furnished housing or a generous housing per diem; Life and AD&D coverage; Optional disability insurance; Travel Reimbursement (travel assignments only); Per Diem meals and incidentals; Travel assignment reimbursements; Free pre-assignment medical screenings; Free license or certification reimbursement; Advanced certification reimbursement; Direct deposit, pay cards, weekly pay, referral bonuses; $1000 bonus for 26-week contracts; Extension benefits; Flexible spending accounts; 24-Hour emergency support service; and an employee discount program.

Randstad Healthcare has been in business over 25 years and they have worked hard to build a reputation based on trust, honesty, and loyalty. They believe in striving for perfection; however, they are aware that no company is perfect. When an issue arises, Randstad Healthcare will take responsibility and work hard to resolve the issue with as little impact as possible to their travelers and to patient care. It's this reputation that has resulted in many of their travelers to choose to continue to work with Randstad for the duration of their travel career, and referring their friends and family to them as well.

At Randstad Healthcare, they work hard to know their candidates.

They also work hard to know their clients. They have a deep understanding of both their candidates and the client's requirements, and are able to align needs, cultures, and work styles to ensure the best match is made. With over 25 years of experience, their industry knowledge takes their travelers to where they want to be in their travel nursing career, whether learning new skills at large teaching hospitals or mentoring the next generation in a local community hospital. They are so committed to helping their travelers to be successful that they mentor their career development from the moment they join their talent network to the moment they walk through their client's doors – working hand-in-hand at every step of the process to gain a deeper understanding of their needs, capabilities, and career goals. As a result, over 70 percent of their candidates have been asked to extend their assignments. But more than that, 100 percent of them are hired for the positions that truly match their skills and aspirations.

For more information, you can contact them at: Randstad Healthcare, 150 Presidential Way, 3rd Floor, Woburn, MA 01801. Phone them at: 800-919-9100, or visit them online at: *www.randstadhealthcare.com.*

~*~

Rise Medical Staffing

Rise Medical Staffing is a small to medium company that places RNs nationwide. Their model is centered on the "nurse first" mentality. They understand that their RNs are the face of Rise and represent their company while on contract. Their recruiters' commission structure is NOT based on margins like a majority of travel companies within the industry. It's based on the number of hours a RN works. In short, it promotes longevity and retention vs. that "one time transaction" where the RN feels like they are being nickled and dimed. They set very competitive pay packages at the company level so the recruiter focus can be on customer service. Miles the recruiter manager states, "Having recruited with Rise for 5 years, I found myself building long lasting relationships which is what their company feels is the cornerstone to their success. We don't sacrifice quality for quantity."

Rise Medical Staffing does have a clinical nurse liaison that is available 24 hours a day. They are a Joint Commission certified company that is looking into belonging to NATHO.

About their recruiter program, Miles states, "As a Recruiter you need to be adaptable. To start, we hire Recruiters that can relate to a large audience and can connect with a variety of individuals. If we find any reoccurring issues with a particular Recruiter (not getting along with RNs, trust issues, etc.) it's a clear sign that the Recruiter isn't a good fit for Rise. However, in the rare occasion that an RN feels their Recruiter simply isn't a good fit, we would redirect the RN to a different Recruiter that best matches what they are looking for. We have every RN complete a survey where the RN can voice their opinion about their Recruiter and other departments (QA, Payroll, Benefits) alike. We always take this feedback serious and will follow up with the RN to ensure we are making changes in areas that need improvement."

Medical insurance is provided through Aetna with offerings of 3 different plans. Vision and Dental insurance is provided by Cypress Insurance. They also provide a 401K with company matching up to 4%.

Other benefits include: Competitive wages for local and travel positions all across the U.S.; Extensive Medical, Dental, Vision Plans; 401k Retirement Savings Account; Free Housing of Tax-Free Stipend – Private, fully furnished, utilities, cable, etc.; $500 Travel Allowance; Tax Advantage Program; Best Referral Program: Refer & Earn; Bonuses, promotions, and more!

I asked Miles, "What makes your company more than just another travel company?" He replied, "Perhaps it sounds cliché, but I think it's all about the people. We started as a very small company and their survival (especially during the recession) was based around people who care about what they do. We want to continue to separate themselves from the pack by pushing for superior customer service. It helps that their company has some of the most competitive pay packages and benefits in the industry. However, it's essential that each employee shares and exhibits their culture and values. Without the right people, we'd be "just another" travel company."

Their recruiters must have the following Rise Medical Staffing Culture of excellence, integrity, collaboration, and fun. This results in Rise Medical Staffing Values: Employees & Clients First; Relationships Matter; Demand Excellence; Be open, honest and constructive; and Act like an owner. Come check them out for yourself – they promise that you will be pleased!

For more information, you can contact them at: 2525 Natomas Park Dr #140, Sacramento, CA 95833. They can be phoned at: 855-747-3562, or visit them online at: *www.risestaffing.com.*

~*~

RN Network

RN Network (RNn) offers 4 to 26 week assignments for RNs, LPNs, Sterile Processors, and ST. They provide nurses in all 50 states as needed. They are a privately held mid-size company. They truly believe this offers the best of both worlds to their clients. They have the backing of a large organization but can operate like a boutique.

Their nurses have one main point of contact, but a full internal team supporting them. They are committed to providing excellent customer service every step of the way. Their recruiters check in with their travelers weekly while on assignment, assuring that they feel a connection with their recruiter and not like a number. They also conduct monthly net promoter surveys to help them continually improve their service and focus on areas that are most important to travelers.

RNn has a Clinical Nurse Liaison that is on staff during business hours, and they have 24/7 emergency support. They are Joint Commission certified and an active member of NATHO. Their President is on the Board of Directors, and their company was one of the founding members.

RNn recruiters spend a lot of time qualifying a traveler during the initial phone call. Their objective is to find out what is most important to the traveler not only in an assignment, but also in an agency and in a recruiter. Their recruiters treat every relationship like a partnership. If during the initial process or assignment the recruiter and traveler do not seem to be a good fit for each other, their leaders will get involved to determine the best next steps, which may include switching to a recruiter that would be a better fit.

They offer excellent medical plans that use the Aetna physician network. They also offer dental and vision insurance. All benefits begin day one of the assignment. They also offer a family and domestic partner coverage. They also offer day one 401K with a company match. Other benefits include: paid Life and AD&D insurance, as well as optional short-term disability, accident insurance, and critical illness insurance.

In addition, they have a benefits team committed to providing a variety of unique benefits that travelers will not find with any other agency. Another amazing benefit is their telephone physician benefit. Nurses can reach a physician 24/7 365 days via this free benefit and receive care and even prescriptions via the telephone.

RN Network is part of CHG Healthcare, they are proud to be ranked #3 on Fortune Magazine's "100 Best Companies to work for in 2013." Their company has great tenure throughout every department, and very little turnover, which allows them to build better relationships with their travelers. They are a company that is built around the idea of "putting people first." They go above and beyond for both their travelers and client facilities to assure that they are providing the best possible service. They are a turn-key establishment; travelers get more personal service and quicker response time for any issues of concerns that may arise. But, the number one thing that makes them more than "just another" travel company is their people, and their passion for what they do.

They start at yes. Their packages are customized and they always seek out of the box solutions to meet our clients/provider's needs. Every provider and situation is different...and they treat them as such.

For more information on RN Network, you can visit them at: 4700 Exchange Ct #125, Boca Raton, FL 33486. You can contact them by phone at: 561-862-0011, or visit them online at: *www.rnnetwork.com.*

~*~

Saratoga Medical Center

Saratoga medical is a medium company that offers assignments nationwide, including Guam and Hawaii.

Saratoga offers a full range of healthcare opportunities across the US. They cover all nursing and advanced nursing specialties, vocational and practical nursing, occupational and physical therapy (and assistants), speech therapy, audiology, physicians, and behavioral health. The military and private sector have called on them for over 30 years for the best healthcare professionals the industry has to offer.

Customer service is very important to them. They consider their employees, nurses included, as important as their clients. Saratoga Medical is accessible to review online through venues such as Indeed, Facebook, and LinkedIn. They also solicit feedback on a regular basis through survey requests and phone calls. Recruiters and Human Resources representatives are reviewed on client and employee satisfaction. They also measure return rates. If they see a high percentage of employees not returning to complete repeat or new assignments they will randomly select one term employees to interview in an effort to determine why and what they could have done to make their experience a better one.

Saratoga has a Clinical Nurse liaison that is available during work hours, and for those that are working night shifts, there is always a dedication overnight point of contact. They are not Joint Commission certified, however they function under strict Government compliance standards, which they must maintain in order to continue performing on contracts. Their compliance and quality is vetted no less than once per month by the military.

Each applicant is first asked to submit an online application, after which a recruitment coordinator reviews the resume in order to ensure a skill set that meets their minimum standards. Once the coordinator vets the resume, she matches the skill set with the recruiter most experienced with that specialty, etc... Home care, ICU, Step Down. he recruitment coordinator will always lead the process with an email and a phone call in which they are told to please contact them if they are not happy with their recruitment representative or the process. Recruiters are evaluated on their complaint resolution rates.

Saratoga Medical provides robust benefits including United Health Insurance and United Dental and Vision. They also provide Life and Short term Disability insurance at no charge. They offer Critical care insurance as a voluntary benefit.

They offer a Nurse only (Voluntary) 401K currently. They also provide sick pay, paid time off (depending on contract type), direct deposit, sign-on bonus, time and a half on all hours worked over eight, dependent care savings plan (Feb 2016), commuter and parking savings plan (Feb 2016), movie, hotel, air, and rental car discount program, entertainment (movies, amusement park, etc.) discount program, unlimited CME, and web courses an online HR portal where employees can request time off, check HR related documents, and a chat feature where employees can speak with an HR representative

Saratoga is different because they aren't just a travel company.

Their perspective ranges from permanent/contract to temporary to travel. Their ability to staff different types of needs make them better able to assist their employees and valued nurses as their needs shift, say from travel back to a contract assignment or vice versa, and because they have the unique ability to serve healthcare workers for a longer period of time they invest much more in (1) finding the right people that meet or exceed minimum standards, (2) developing a real and meaningful relationship with each one, and (3) offering a benefits package that is geared to a longer term relationship. They think beyond 13 weeks.

They started from a Government contracting organization and now services travel and private clients across the US. They are dedicated to the military clients and to the level of excellence they expect. This dedication to quality transfers into everything they do including their travel nursing division. You can expect customer service from day one and to feel that you are part of a team. They go the extra mile to make sure that your needs and careers goals are met.

For more information, you can visit them at: 16 West 32nd Street, New York, NY 10001. You can also contact them by phone at: (212) 213-2520, or visit their website at: *www.saratogamed.com.*

~*~

Soliant Health

Soliant Health offers opportunities in the following specialties: RN, School Nurse, Physician Assistant, Nurse Practitioner, CST, PT, OT, SLP, Physician, Pharmacist, Pharmacy Technician, and Healthcare IT. They offer full-time, part-time, travel, and per diem assignments nationwide. They are considered a small company that operates as part of Adecco Group North America, a larger company that is publicly traded on the stock market.

As a Soliant healthcare professional, you'll enjoy a personal relationship with a recruiter who is as passionate about your career as you are. Your recruiter works tirelessly to match your personal goals, interests, strengths and professional aspirations with the right job, in the right place. But it doesn't stop there. Your recruiter is always with you, available for assistance, advice, or simply an understanding ear on which you can always count.

They do have a clinical nurse liaison who is a nurse practitioner and available during normal business hours. Although they are Joint Commission certified, they do not belong to NATHO.

Soliant recruiters are trained to operate with nursing candidates' career goals in mind. In any event that a recruiter and a nurse are not a good fit, a Soliant Nursing Division manager will step in to help find a resolution.

They provide comprehensive health insurance for nursing professionals and their families. Unlike some recruiting companies, their associates receive the same great insurance options as their employee staff.

As a nursing professional through Soliant Health, nurses are eligible and encouraged to join theirs. Nurses can make regular, easy contributions through payroll deductions. And nurses also receive matching contributions from them. Choose from a variety of safe investment choices.

- Weekly Paychecks. Unlike other staffing companies, Soliant Health, pays nurses weekly, not every two weeks or every month. Every Friday their nurses receive a paper check or, if they prefer, direct deposit.
- Free Travel. When nurses travel from job to job, they have enough to do without making (and paying for) their own travel arrangements. So Soliant travel specialists handle those details for its travel nurses.
- Custom Housing. their travel nurses don't have to search for places to live or put down rent deposits when they mobilize to a new city. Soliant Health provides custom housing that's comfortable, safe, secure and close to their work assignment in some of the nicest parts of town.
- Licensing Assistance. State licensing requirements are complicated, and they vary from one state to another. Soliant Health has specialists who help nurses navigate this licensing maze, so they can focus on what they do best.

It's this consistent, one-on-one attention that sets Soliant Health apart from other healthcare staffing agencies. Well, this and the fact that they go the distance for their healthcare professionals, taking care of every last detail – travel plans, housing and scheduling – so you can focus on your job, and yourself!

As a nursing professional with Soliant Health, nurses receive a benefit package that combines traditional employee benefits with many that are innovative. These benefits don't just help their nurses excel in their job performance, they support and enhance their lives on and off the job. They see that as a win-win proposition. That's how they built their reputation for attracting the best nursing professionals in the industry.

For more information, you can visit them here: 979 Lakeside Pkwy, Tucker, GA 30084. They can also be phoned at: 800.849.5502, or you can visit their website at: *www.soliant.com.*

~*~

Springboard Healthcare

SpringBoard Healthcare supplies RN, RT, RCIS, RCES, and IBHRE's for cardiology assignments. They have nationwide travel assignments along with a local market per diem opportunities in Southern California.

SpringBoard is a consulting, education and talent acquisition partner for leading hospitals and healthcare organizations that are looking to develop, optimize or expand their cardiovascular service lines. Established in 2002, SpringBoard is staffed by industry experts and thought leaders that are dedicated to staying up-to-date on that latest advancements and requirements in this rapidly growing field. SpringBoard works with some of the most prestigious institutions across the nation to provide best-in-class training programs, top-tier talent and strategic consulting services. The company's annual wage survey is also considered the gold standard in the industry for compensation benchmarks.

SpringBoard is a small niche company whose top priority is to develop trusting long lasting relationships with their travelers. At SpringBoard that means that within their company they adhere to their core values of: Trust, Accountability, Urgency and Credibility. In addition, they are niche focused which means, unlike most other companies, they understand your area of expertise better than their competition. Finally, their Relationship Managers are easily accessible 7 days a week.

They are Joint Commission certified, and they have an RN educator that serves as their nurse liaison. Their relationship managers receive performance evaluations and their direct supervisor does sporadic audit calls with clinical staff.

When it comes to benefits, they offer 2 plans from Aetna with vision, dental, and disability. SpringBoard also provides a 401k with numerous options matched at the company discretion. They also have an online payroll portal, free lunch or dinner if you go see them in Phoenix, and many opportunities to grow into other divisions such as training, or consulting. Differentiators include SpringBoard niche focus, market tools that provide insight and training in the form of their Salary Survey, and training curriculum to name a few.

Clinical professionals have many choices which is fantastic. If you are looking for a partner for a long term relationship not just a recruiter SpringBoard would like to talk to you. They have deep relationships nationwide in cardiovascular medicine.

You can visit them at: 6910 E. Chauncey Lane, Suite 150, Phoenix, AZ 85054. You can contact them by phone at: 866-465-6286, or visit them online at: *springboardhealthcare.com.*

~*~

Sunbelt Staffing

Sunbelt Staffing offers nursing, therapy, advanced practice, and school-based healthcare career opportunities nationwide.

Sunbelt is a small company that is not publicly traded on the stock market. Although they are Joint Commission certified, they do not belong to NATHO. They have a clinical nurse liaison during business hours.

They make sure that their nurses are number one through established relationships with facilities across the country, Sunbelt helps nurses find their perfect fit. For those wishing to add some diversity and adventure to their career, the Sunbelt travel program is just what the nurse ordered.

At Sunbelt, they work hard to find each and every nurse a position that matches both their specialty and their specific requirements. Since they have positions opening and closing every day, the best way to see what they have available for your chosen specialty is to speak with one of their recruiters. Their recruiters will always have the most up-to-date opportunities and will work to ensure that you find an assignment that suits your unique needs.

Their insurance coverage consist of: major medical, surgical and prescription drug coverage; Dental insurance; Vision plan; Group life insurance; and Liability insurance. Other benefits include: Virtual Instant Paycheck (V.I.P.) Card – Experience the ultimate in convenience when it comes to getting paid. Their V.I.P. card can provide you with simple, immediate ATM access to all of your pay, bonuses, and reimbursements worldwide. After all, it's your money. Shouldn't you be able to access it where and when you need it?

At Sunbelt Staffing, they take pride in caring for all of their healthcare professionals. That means providing plenty of perks and benefits in addition to the highest paying opportunities the nursing industry has to offer. When you are a part of the Sunbelt team, you will earn more than just a paycheck.

Sunbelt Cares is a colleague-created initiatives that aims to invest resources back into every community they and their nurses are in. They encourage travel nurses to support environmental and social causes as part of Sunbelt Cares. At Sunbelt, a job well done means happy people, who are not only engaged in their work but in their communities too.

For more information, you can visit them at: 3687 Tampa Rd. Ste. 200, Oldsmar, FL 34677. You can phone them at: 813-471-0152, or visit them online at: *www.sunbeltstaffing.com.*

~*~

TaleMed

TaleMed offers travel assignments for RN's, Allied Health, and P.T. These range from 8 weeks, 13 weeks, and 26 weeks.

TaleMed was founded upon dedication to strong moral and ethical principles. They take the time to make sure all Healthcare Professionals who choose to travel with TaleMed receive the attention they deserve and are properly educated about the industry, as a whole, and every detail about the positions they accept. TaleMed's processes to properly screen validate, and match talented healthcare professionals to assignments in all 50 states is backed by a talented staff with in-depth knowledge of the Healthcare Travel industry. Along with their top-notch customer service, they have exceptional benefits including medical/prescription offered through United Healthcare and Dental and optional Vision coverage offered through Guardian and Davis Vision. Just recently they have also added a 401K program!

TaleMed's inner office culture is one that constantly re-imagines proven methodologies to keep up with the times, provides an environment of open communication, fosters teamwork, encourages honesty, and acts responsibly. Every TaleMed employee is encouraged to create "Win-Win" situations in every relationship.

TaleMed, LLC began operations in March of 2006 in Loveland, OH. Today, TaleMed has clients in all 50 states, and boasts a 95% retention rating for all of their employees. In September of 2007, TaleMed received the Gold Seal of Approval for Healthcare Staffing by The Joint Commission. In 2016 they were rated as one of the Best Staffing Firms to work for. Their work serves Healthcare professionals, hospitals, and most importantly the patients. TaleMed assignments in public and private facilities, including: acute care hospitals, trauma centers and community hospitals. Work with them and you will receive the quality or customer service and attention to detail that is required for success.

For more information, you can find them at: 6279 Tri-Ridge Blvd, Suite 110, Loveland, OH 45140. You can also phone them at: 800-494-0087, or visit them online at: *www.talemed.com.*

~*~

Tailored Healthcare Staffing

Tailored Healthcare Staffing (THS) is a medium sized company that places RNs and Surgical Techs throughout the nation.

THS understands that their nurses are their number one asset. The nurses are the reason they are in business! Travelers receive 24/7 personal attention from their staff. THS offers the benefits of larger companies while receiving the personalized attention of smaller ones. Their recruiters are exceptional career coaches who are dedicated and easily accessible. They have dedicated credentialing and housing departments as well who work with each nurse individually to make sure every assignment goes smoothly. They treat their travel professionals just as they do their internal staff. That's why THS travel nurses are entitled to the same industry leading benefits, including 1st day platinum level medical insurance, 401k with match, paid state licensure, and their Corporate Rewards Program. They are also a member of NATHO.

Their goal is to provide nurses with a tailored traveling experience over the course of many successful and fulfilling assignments. The nurse-recruiter relationship is at the core of this goal. A testament to their success in this area is their high rate of assignment extensions, nurses who have been traveling with them for many years, and their large number of referrals from nurses who love working with their recruiters.

Additionally, they are always looking for feedback from their travelers. If ever an issue arises, they are here to listen and to fix the problem.

THS offers first day platinum level medical insurance from Anthem Blue Cross Blue Shield for $18 per week. Tailored Healthcare makes large contributions so they can offer a high quality plan at low rates. They offer vision, dental, and life insurance as well. Internal employees receive the same high quality insurance options as their travelers.

They offer a 401k plan with company match of 10% of the first 6% of contributions. Employees have their choice of either traditional pre-tax or post-tax Roth plans. They have a large selection of funds to choose from so that travelers can meet their retirement goals.

Weekly pay and direct deposit, customized housing options for travelers, their families and pets, travel reimbursement, paid state licensure, dedicated recruiters with after-hour call availability, professional liability insurance, Corporate Rewards Program covering car rentals, airfare, etc., financial support for CEUs, choice of company paid housing or housing stipends, tax advantage pay packages with per diems or fully taxable pay packages, assignments across the country in both big cities and rural areas, Referral Bonuses, Extension Bonuses, Completion Bonuses, and Holiday Bonuses.

Incredible People – The culture at THS is unrivaled. Their recruiters are great people, full of energy, personality and insight on the RN travel market. They're not just recruiters, they're exceptional career coaches, if you'd like them to be.

They're Social – They're not just on social media, they're actively engaging nearly 30,000 nurses every day on their Facebook and Twitter pages! While many use these platforms to pedal jobs, they are writing unique industry content and sharing the best nursing stories and memes on the Internet!

Platinum Level Benefits – Every agency has benefits. At THS, they try to provide their nurses with the best options on the market, like low-cost platinum level health insurance starting on day one of your assignment. A 401k retirement plan with employer match tops off an unbeatable package.

Joint Commission Certification – Joint Commission accreditation and certification is recognized nationwide as a symbol of quality that reflects an organization's commitment to meeting certain performance standards. At their last re-certification, they were honored to receive a perfect score with no deficiencies. This is a reflection of their efforts to employee the highest quality standards in the industry.

You'll Make and Save Lots of Money – Aside from the high pay you expect, Tailored Healthcare offers may ways to help nurses save including financial support to continue education (CEU), paid state licensure, travel reimbursement, and access to their corporate rewards program discounts on car rentals, airfare and everyday purchases.

For more information, you can contact them at: 1700 Madison Road, Suite 100, Cincinnati, OH 45206. They can be reached by phone at: 800-927-5918, or visit them on the web at: *www.thstravel.com.*

The Right Solutions

The Right Solutions staffs RNs, LPNs, and CSTs. They are a small company that was founded by and owned by Diana Wright, RN. Staffing is their core business and they offer assignments nationwide at both large city hospitals and small critical access hospitals. They also staff for Indian Health Services (HIS) and Veterans Administration (VA) facilities.

With a motto of, "You're a nurse, not a number," the focus of their entire team is treating you as an individual instead of a number. They do extensive training and specialization with all team members and departments to ensure everyone is laser-focused on treating each nurse as an individual. Every nurse is unique and has unique needs. It is their privilege to recognize and address these needs on an individual basis. They encourage their recruiters to get to know each nurse as an individual to understand individual needs. They also do extensive training on communication and behavioral understanding. This allows recruiters to communicate in the best way possible. If on a rare occasion a recruiter and nurse aren't a fit, they will change recruiters at the nurse's discretion.

The Right Solutions (TRS) was one of the first healthcare staffing agencies to be accredited by The Joint Commission. They also belong to NATHO and actively engage for consistent staffing practices amongst agencies.

Their benefits include Blue Cross/Blue Shield, vision, dental, life and short-term disability. They also offer an IRA with 50% company match. TRS specialized support departments whose focus is to be an expert in their area. Housing choices allow you to choose and determine the cost and location of housing.

When asked what makes them different, CEO, Caleb English stated, "Work for a company whose founder wore scrubs, not a suit. Experience the difference when your company has walked a mile in your shoes. You comfort and restore the lives of patients every day, it's time you join a team who does the same for you."

For more information you can contact them at PO Box 595, Tontitown, AR 72770. They can also be reached by phone at: 888-987-8233 or visit their website at: *www.therightsolutions.com.*

~*~

Total Med Staffing

TotalMed offers flexible staffing solutions such as: per diem, local contract, travel nursing, contract-to-hire, and direct placement. They offer assignments for RNs, CSTs, PTs, OTs, and various other allied specialties. They are Joint Commission certified, and they belong to NATHO.

They have assignments in all 50 states and pride themselves on the quality of relationships they have with their direct clients. TotalMed Staffing is a medium-sized, minority-owned and privately owned healthcare staffing agency. However, TotalMed is committed to their intimate customer service that allowed them to grow from a small company to where they are now.

TotalMed's success relies on its ability to reflect and evolve, not only competitively but also in their relationships. Apart from the licensing, background checks, phone screens, and contract agreements that are a part of every day in the office, recruiters spend their time reaching out to their nurses to ensure they are being taken care of. This process is reciprocated with quarterly evaluations in which healthcare professionals are invited to complete surveys and provide feedback on their experience with TotalMed. This exchange is very important as it gives TotalMed the opportunity to evaluate these processes as a whole in order to improve the overall experience with current and future employees.

They remain open after its doors close. Their recruiters are always just a phone call away and they have a Clinical Nurse Liaison and an after-hours contact available 24/7/365 to both clients and healthcare professionals. Their attentiveness and willing to lend an ear is what separates them from other staffing agencies and has earned them multiple awards.

TotalMed Staffing doesn't just build contracts, they build relationships by catering to their nurses' needs and concerns on a daily basis. Compatibility is an important aspect of job placement and their recruiters use all of their resources to effectively place nurses in locations they are going to be comfortable for their travel assignments. By taking into account nurses' family lives, preferences, needs, and abilities the recruiters will compete to find the nurses the best match.

Their company's various benefits and insurance policies for full time employees are what promote loyalty and unity in their company. Immediate active health insurance is offered through United Healthcare Group and will accommodate individual needs of employees. United Healthcare Group offers two plans in addition to a Benefits Coordinator that consults with each applicant regarding their program and their options. They will walk all applicants through their procedures to ensure their satisfaction with all available options.

Employees can also enroll in a substantial 401K program on their first day. Administered by Fidelity the 401K program compensates fifty cents for every dollar up to 6% deferred. In addition to insurance, TotalMed offers several plans regarding dental, vision, cancer, accident, disability, and other alternatives. They also offer a flexible spending plan which allows employees to defer dollars pre-taxed to compensate reimbursable medical or dependent care expenses. All employees who elect to participate in benefits receive a $10,000 company paid life insurance plan and short-term disability coverage. A free employee assistance program is a part of the package purposed for contributing to the welfare of all employees.

TotalMed Staffing is a family that cares like no other when it comes to working with both local and travel nurses. TotalMed Nurses feel part of the TotalMed "family" and more like internal employees than contractors. Their niche of offering customer focused people solutions allows to achieve their core focus of improving lives.

For more information on TotalMed Staffing you can visit them at: 10 East College Ave., Suite 300, Appleton, WI 54911. You can contact them at: 866-288-8001, or visit them online at: *www.totalmedstaffing.com.*

~*~

The Quest Group

The Quest Group consistently earns a reputation for top talent, top rates, superior benefits, lucrative bonus programs, and much more.

They are seeking talented, experienced healthcare professionals for rewarding travel, local and per diem assignments in major cities throughout the United States. They are a top supplier of temporary and permanent healthcare services for all nursing and allied specialties. They are a moderately sized company, which staffs healthcare professionals throughout the United States.

They have achieved the Gold Seal of Approval for health care staffing services from The Joint Commission. Quest Group recently underwent an on-site review of its compliance with national standards addressing how staffing firms determine the qualifications and competency of their staff, how they place their staff, and how they monitor staff's performance. They also have a Clinical Nurse Liaison that is available 24/7.

The Quest Group spends time getting to know their nurses and their loved ones. They understand that you are away from your closest friends and family for a long period of time. For that reason they are available 24/7 to speak with you. Call them at home or on the weekend if you have a problem or just want to talk! They are here for you!

They have learned over the years that nurses and recruiters can love each other or not really love each other! For that reason they have created the 30-day recruiter return policy. If your recruiter does not do everything in their power to help you and create time for you then you may simply ask for a better fit and they will find a recruiter that matches with your needs and wants.

The Quest Group knows the importance of taking care of its employees and their families. With this in mind, The Quest Group has put together an outstanding benefits package that is offered to their employees. This package includes: Health Insurance–BlueCross/BlueShield health insurance along with vision and dental insurance; a 401K; Competitive Pay–The Quest Group strives to get their staff the highest pay rates possible at all of their contracted facilities; Benefits–They are pleased to offer to all their employees' medical benefits that can be tailored to you and your family's needs, and new employees have 30 days from the date of hire to enroll for health benefits; 24/7 Support for Nurses–The Quest Group office hours are 8 am to 5 pm – Monday through Friday. Also, a Quest Group representative is available on-call after hours and on weekends to assist you with any needs; Malpractice Insurance–They carry malpractice, liability, and worker's compensation insurance on all their staff and employees; Direct Deposit–You can choose to have your pay direct deposited into your checking and/or savings account for your convenience; Flexible Schedules–The Quest Group gives you total control over your work schedule. You choose which days and how many hours you want to work; Scheduling Control–They use TSS Scheduling software to give you 24/7 access to your work schedule; and Weekly Paychecks–The Quest Group pays all its employees on a weekly basis. Their work week runs Sunday through Saturday and pay day is every Friday. You can log into ADP IPay at www.Portal.ADP.com to view your pay statements and other personal Information.

What makes The Quest Group more than "just another" travel company? (1) Their Vision! The Quest Group Continually Strives To Be the Leader – Not the Biggest, But the Best. The Leader in Rewards and Recognition for their Associates; The Leader In Opportunity To Grow And Learn; The Leader In The Quality Of their Relationships and Treatment Of Others; The Leader In The Quality Of Patient Care We Deliver; The Leader In The Value We Deliver To their Clients; and The Leader In Attitude And Excellence In Service. (2) Their Guiding

Values And Principles. They recognize that they are most effective as a team and they continually strive to strengthen their relationships with each other and their customers. They strive to lead by example. They pledge to perform with honesty, integrity and excellence in all they do. They will be ever alert to improve their skills and the quality of patient care. They view learning as a lifelong commitment. They strive for the highest standards of clinical practice. At The Quest Group you will definitely be treated like family!

For more information, you can contact them at: 9300 Wade Blvd, Frisco, TX 75035. You can phone them at: 469-888-4900, or visit them online here: *questgroupstaffing.com.*

~*~

Travel Nurse across America

At Travel Nurse across America (TNAA) they focus on exceeding expectations and take pride in the fact that they provide highly personalized service and accommodate each nurse's unique needs and plans.

They specialize in 8 to 26 week travel assignments for registered nurses. The typical assignment is 13 weeks. They place a high value on individual attention, respect, and a genuine commitment to every nurse they work with. Their entire staff builds positive, long-lasting connections with the travel nurses they serve.

Travel Nurse across America is a medium-sized company who places nurses all over the United States, but do not currently offer international assignments. Being a medium sized company allows them access to a wide array of clients while, at the same time, helps them stay nimble and able to respond quickly to changes in the marketplace. Because they are not a huge organization, their recruiters are able to spend time getting to know the nurses they work with, thereby providing highly personalized service. They have representatives on call 24/7/365 so that you can reach someone who has the authority to address any issues that might arise while you are on assignment. After-hours calls are answered by a live person so that you receive immediate attention. Typically the on-board process takes between two and four weeks, based on both the hospital and nurses' needs, desires, and readiness. If a traveler is truly ready to go, and the hospital is ready to receive, they can take a nurse from acceptance of application to their first day on the job in less than two weeks.

They offer an extremely competitive benefit package, including: Your Way Is Paid: They pay all costs associated with getting the licenses and certifications you need for the travel assignment you've accepted. They also arrange and pay for any physical examinations and immunizations you may need to start working. Guaranteed pay: If you've contracted to work 36 or 40 hours each week and the hospital census drops to the point that you're not needed for a day, don't worry. If your paycheck is going to be less than normal due to low census, they'll make up the difference. Tax-Advantage: They'll help you understand whether you qualify for their tax-advantage program and, if you do, leverage the use of it. Travel Money: They reimburse for up to $1,000 in expenses for you to get to your assignment. How you choose to travel is up to you. If you're working close to home and don't need travel expense money they roll what they would have reimbursed into a higher hourly pay rate. Housing: They offer several housing options to fit their nurse's individual needs. You can chose from high-quality, furnished, private, company provided housing with 100% of the utilities paid. Or, you can opt for a housing subsidy and use their Easy Stay program. With Easy Stay you receive the full benefit of your housing subsidy while a TNAA housing specialist helps you through every step of setting up your new living space! Sick Leave: Travel Nurse across America is proud to offer paid sick leave to all of their travel nurses. Sick leave begins accruing from your first day, and you're eligible to use it after 90 days of employment. If you take additional assignments with TNAA within a one-year period, you can take advantage of their carryover policy and keep the unused time you've accrued. Though you may only work for a hospital on a temporary basis, you're a permanent part of the TNAA team, and they always have your needs in mind. Insurance: Their travelers are covered from day 1! They offer a low-deductible PPO plan through United Healthcare that covers doctor visits, wellness exams, diagnostic tests, prescription medications, and hospitalization. TNAA pays 100% of their traveler's premium and spouse and/or children can be added at a low cost. Their comprehensive insurance package also offers dental insurance through Delta Dental and liability. Their insurance are as good as you'll find anywhere in the industry.

Other benefits include: Free Continuing Education. When you travel with us, you have access to more than 400 CE courses online through CE Direct. There is no limit on the number of courses you can take. Multiple Bonus Opportunities: They offer all of the usual sign on, completion, extension, and referral bonus plans, but their unique extra shift bonus is the one that nurses seem to love the most. If a hospital offers you extra shifts and you accept, you get a bonus in additional to the usual extra pay you earn. Loyalty Bonus program: This unique program allows you to earn points for every hour you work and redeem those points for cash anytime you're on assignment with them. There is no limit to the number of points you can earn and you can use them for anything – home improvements, holiday shopping, to build up your rainy day fund, to tap into when you miss work due to illness, or to give yourself a paid vacation. Referral Bonus: Their Referral Bonus plan is different from other firms. When you refer a colleague who works with them for at least eight weeks, you get $500 – half up front and half when they complete their assignment. Assignment Benefits Summary: For each assignment you're considering with Travel Nurse across America you'll receive a one-page document that spells out your hourly rate, applicable taxes, benefits, and your net take home pay, both weekly and for the length of the assignment. JobWatch: This one-of-a-kind program notifies you immediately by email or text message when a job you've been waiting for becomes available.

Travel Nurse across America consistently hear from their nurses that their obvious focus on personal attention is the single most important reason for their enduring loyalty to TNAA. They don't take that loyalty for granted and they're always looking for new and better ways to make their nurses feel like they are part of their family. They have both a Clinical Nurse Liaison and a Director or Nursing who are available 24/7.

They are Joint Commission Certified and have been awarded a Gold Seal of Approval. Meeting high quality standards and adhering to the most stringent clinical and ethical criteria in the industry is very important to them. They have been a member of NATHO since its inception.

Travel Nurse across America screen and hire their internal recruiters based on their experience and ability to understand what nurses want and need. It almost never happens, but if a travel nurse ever feels that a recruiter is not a good match for them they will happily assign them to someone else within the firm.

Their travelers are covered from day 1 with a quality PPO! They offer a low-deductible plan through United Healthcare that covers doctor visits, wellness exams, diagnostic tests, prescription medications, and hospitalization. TNAA pays 100% of their traveler's premium and spouse and/or children can be added at a low cost. Their comprehensive insurance package also offers dental insurance through Delta Dental and liability. Their insurance are as good as you'll find anywhere in the industry.

They don't offer a 401K at this time. Instead, they have several unique bonus programs that nurses can participate in to boost their income and contribute all or part of that bonus money to their own personal retirement plan.

Call them to talk about what you want from your travel nursing career. They will listen and you will be happy you made the connection – they promise.

For more information, you can contact them at: 5020 Northshore Dr., Suite 2, North Little Rock, AR 72118. You may contact them by phone at: 800-240-2526, or visit their website at: *www.nurse.tv*.

~*~

Trinity Healthcare Staffing Group

Trinity Healthcare Staffing Group offers travel assignments to various specialties of healthcare professionals that typically range in duration from 8 to 13 weeks.

Longer or shorter assignments can be negotiated. Also, a traveler typically has the option of renewing the assignment or rolling into a new assignment. Per Diem shifts are also available. Travel assignments are offered nationwide, including Alaska and Hawaii. There are a variety of settings to include teaching hospitals, rural facilities, long term care, clinics, and rehab facilities. Assignments are chosen based on skills, specialties, certifications, and experience.

Trinity Healthcare Staffing Group is a medium sized company that offers large company rates and benefits. Once the lead or referral is made and a recruiter is assigned and makes contact with a nurse, the process is initiated to create that relationship. They never refer to their nurses as numbers but always by name. As the nurse goes through the application, credentialing and submittal processes, the nurse will become familiar with many of the internal staff apart from the recruiter as well (Placement Specialist, QA, Payroll, Housing, CNO, etc.). Each contact makes the nurse feel welcome and assists with helping in the placement process. The recruiter provides the nurse with his or her contact phone number and email address so that the nurse may have 24/7 access. There is also after hour support staff on call in case the nurse has questions or issues. They also have a Clinical Nurse Liaison who is also available 24 hours a day, 7 days a week. Trinity has been Joint Commission certified since 2006, and is a member of NATHO.

Trinity Healthcare Staffing Group helps a nurse to get his/her travel career headed in a positive direction by matching not only with the right job order but with the right recruiter. Connecting the professional with an employment opportunity that will give them a chance to utilize his/her specific skills and training to serve patients in a variety of different types of medical facilities is the job of the recruiter. It is also the role of the recruiter to create and build a relationship with the professional. Their goal is to help find the ideal position to meet the individual needs of each traveler. They take care of all of the ground work for securing a position, even locating housing if needed, so that the professional can focus on providing an exceptional level of care. Although rarely occurring, there are times when a switch in recruiter and/or nurse is requested and this is handled without any negativity among staff.

Trinity Healthcare provides Blue Cross insurance, as well as vision, dental, life and professional liability. Benefits for dependents are also available and can be payroll deducted. Trinity also has a great 401K retirement plan. Other benefits include full reimbursement for licensure fees once the assignment is started. Trinity also will reimburse for cost of continuing education that is specific to your clinical specialty for current travelers with prior approval. Free CEUs are also offered. Travel reimbursement is available and depends on the package selected, and is completely tax-free. Trinity also offers free housing so you pay nothing for your housing or furniture.

What's different about Trinity? Everything! Trinity Healthcare is owned and operated by a former traveling nurse, and their internal staff consists of nurses and other professionals who have been there, done that. The Recruiter and/or support staff are always available, day or night, 24/7 ensuring the Traveler never gets left stranded away from home without support. Trinity offers some of the highest compensation plans in the industry. Most importantly, they operate according to their core mission and values, meaning, "We'll do what we say we'll do." They have many longstanding relationships with clients, vendors, and employees to prove their commitment to being one of the best staffing companies in the industry.

Trinity Healthcare was started by a traveling nurse who struggled with the inconsistencies and disorganization that defined the profession Often showing up to bewildered looks instead of secured housing. Paychecks that rarely landed on time, and when they did, routinely were inaccurate. It is because of these experiences that makes Trinity very different from other travel companies. "We do what we say we'll do." Bottom-line. No questions asked. How simple is that? You will not find another company that will give you the support, security and respect that Trinity provides each and every travel nurse.

For more information, you can contact them at: 1834 Sally Hill Farms Blvd, Florence, SC 29501. You can phone them at: 877-417-9507, or visit them online at: *www.trinityhsg.com.*

~*~

Trustaff

Trustaff offers travel opportunities for nurses, therapists, pharmacists, and allied healthcare professionals all across the country.

They work with professionals of all types, in every specialty, and leverages their extensive knowledge of the healthcare industry to help deliver the best travel experience possible and grow their travelers' careers.

Trustaff is a mid-sized, privately-owned company that specializes in travel, but also offers per diem and permanent placement nationwide. Trustaff prides themselves on the personal relationships they develop with each traveler year after year. With so much of their business built on trust, they make the satisfaction of their travelers their number one priority. Each potential traveler is matched with a dedicated career specialist who takes the time to listen and learn their specific needs, goals, and personal preferences. Once a travel contract has been accepted, Trustaff maintains regular contact and provides support to all of their travelers throughout the assignment and often years into the future. Trustaff's devoted team of Nurse Advocates is also available to their travelers for additional assistance in the event their career specialist is busy assisting another traveler. Trustaff knows healthcare is a 24/7 operation, so they too provide 24/7/365 support. Should a traveler need immediate assistance after hours, they can call the support line to be directed to a live member of Trustaff's team at any time.

Trustaff has been certified by The Joint Commission, is a member of NATHO, and is committed to abiding by and furthering ethical business practices in the travel industry. Trustaff intends on providing great service, maintaining HIPAA compliance, and pursuing continuous excellence in healthcare staffing.

Trustaff offers a wide range of healthcare plans – skip the wait with their day-one insurance program, or select your level of coverage through United Healthcare's coverage plans. Plans cover medical, dental, and vision for each employee as well as additional family members and dependents. Your benefits can continue seamlessly even when you change assignments, as long as you don't have a break between assignments longer than 28 days. Trustaff employees are also eligible to make contributions to a 401k savings account managed by USB, upon taking their first assignment. After completion of one year of employment and at least 1,000 hours of work, Trustaff will match your contributions at 50%, up to the first 4% of contributions. Trustaff's unique paid time off (PTO) program is one of their traveler's favorite perks. The more assignments you complete, the more days you earn! In addition to their industry-leading compensation, benefits packages, and personal service, Trustaff offers all employees weekly direct deposit, holiday pay, guaranteed hours, licensure reimbursement, housing assistance, and loyalty, referral, and sign-on bonuses.

Trustaff recognizes that traveling is more than just a job; it's an experience. When you're out in an unfamiliar location, away from family and friends, it makes a big difference to have someone on your side that knows the ins and outs of the business. Trustaff makes their best effort to go above and beyond to ensure their travelers' needs are being met and to make their experience traveling a positive one. The personal relationships they develop with their travelers truly put Trustaff a touch above the rest.

To find out more information, you can contact them at: 4270

Glendale-Milford Road, Cincinnati, OH 45242. You can phone them at: 877-880-0346, or visit them online at: *www.trustafftravel.com.*

~*~

United Staffing Solutions Inc.

"United Staffing Serves one nurse and one client with excellence and repeat that thousands of times."

United Staffing is a medium Premier Travel RN Provider which has nationwide assignments all 50 states. They are a Joint Commission Certified company that has a clinical liaison available 24/7 for support to their nurses, clients and internal staff.

United Staffing has an extensive interview process to uncover exactly what their nurses are looking for. Once they understand what the nurses' needs and wants are they work tirelessly to provide them with jobs that are a perfect fit. They are huge believers in a balanced approach to business and life.

They have a plethora of options for Medical, Dental, and Vision. They provide all of these benefits through California Choice. Other benefits include 401k (without match), top industry pay, great customer service, nationwide jobs, and company provided housing.

United Staffing is built around travel nurses and in an age when customer service often gets overlooked we strive to provide the best service possible to all of our nurses, clients and corporate employees.

For more information, you can contact them at: 12069 Jefferson Blvd, Culver City, CA 90230. You can also phone them at: 888-311-0000, or visit them online at: *www.ussinurses.com.*

~*~

Voyage Solutions

Voyage Solutions has opportunities for RNs PTs, OTs, SLPs, CSTs, RT, Diagnostic Imaging, and occasionally medical device opportunities in all 50 states.

They are a medium sized company that is not publicly traded. One thing that makes them different is that their President of operations makes sure to speak to every Healthcare Provider prior to starting any assignment with Voyage. They believe that it is very important to speak to each individual on a phone call as too much can be improperly communicated by text or by email.

Voyage has a clinical liaison available to discuss clinical issues as needed. They are JCAHO certified but we are not NATHO – they are very rigorous with their JCAHO standards.

If there is ever an issue with a recruiter/candidate "fit", their president of operations will contact the candidate and take over the relationship until such time as a more suitable match can be made.

For 2015/2016 they have United Healthcare and utilize a different insurance company for their dental/vision. They make every effort to meet the needs of the individual.

Voyage has been and will always be fully matched up to 3% of income and they offer fully vested funds from day one of participation in their 401k program. Their fundamental emphasis for this level of commitment to their employees is that they are helping to improve quality of life.

They have a large portfolio of benefits that are additionally available through their Payroll Company. Discounted theme parks, car rentals, hotel stays, and movie tickets are just a few of the perks.

Voyage guarantees their pay – meaning that they will not be beat by any other staffing firm for the same job. Their size means that they are fully funded and also that they can be nimble to change as needed to accommodate the individual.

Voyage has a very simple goal to be the most respected firm in the business. They know every employee and treat all of them with the respect that they have earned and deserve.

If you have any question about the difference in working with Voyage. We encourage you to call a few companies first, and then call them. Their systems are simple; their staff are friendly; their pay is excellent; their benefits cannot be matched; and they will do whatever it takes to be the best travel experience possible.

For more information, you can find them at: 4566 Orange Blvd Suite 1006, Sanford, FL 32771. You can also phone them at: 800-798-6035, or visit them online at: *www.voyagesolutions.com.*

Appendix A

Traveling Healthcare Resources

Highway Hypodermics®, LLC – The home of this book series. It is the mission of the Highway Hypodermics® website to provide quality and up to date information to travel nurses around the world to assist them in finding the adventure of a lifetime. It is our mission to bridge the gap between traveling nurses and travel nurse companies. Only by education on how to be a quality traveling nurse and how to be a traveling company with great integrity can we change the image of both sides. www.highwayhypodermics.com

Highway Hypodermics: Travel Company Profiles – There are over 400 travel nursing companies out there that place nurses in all 50 states. This is by far the biggest list of travel nursing company profiles available on the Internet. Find a few that interest you and then check out who has the best benefits! http://highwayhypodermics.com/wp/travel-company-information/travel-company-profiles/

Highway Hypodermics Travel Company Benefits – With so many travel companies out there, how is a nurse to pick the best one? This chart was made to assist you find the right travel nursing company for YOU! This list is made up of the top 21 benefits that traveling professionals expressed knowing about a travel company. http://ww.highwayhypodermics.com/wp/travel-company-information/travel-company-benefits/

Highway Hypodermics: Travel Company Evaluations – The first question I'm asked by newbies is, "Who is the best travel nursing company?" Don't take my personal opinion! Visit the website to find over 1400 evaluations from travel nurses out there on the road. These are updated every month; therefore the list keeps on growing astronomically. http://highwayhypodermics.com/wp/travel-company-information/travel-company-evaluations/

Highway Hypodermics: Top Ten Travel Companies – A list of the top travel nursing companies that is renewed every January. The requirements of this reward include: (1) Must have at least 20 company evaluations. (2) Must have an updated list of benefits, and (3) Must have an updated company profile. This is a great place to start your search for your perfect company! http://highwayhypodermics.com/wp/travel-company-information/top-ten-travel-companies/

Highway Hypodermics: Travel Nursing Hospital Evaluations – This will be the accumulation of data from all forms filled out. The purpose of this list is for the travel nurse a better look at hospitals around the country. This is an accumulation of all nursing data acquired through our survey. http://highwayhypodermics.com/wp/travel-nursing-information/hospital-evaluations/

Highway Hypodermics: Free Travel Nursing Forms – Wondering what to ask the hospital during an interview? There are quite a few lists out there, but this is my personal one that I formulated to fit my needs. You are free to take it and pass it around to other travel nurses also! Forms include: (1) Questions For Hospital, (2) Questions For Travel Agency, and (3) City/Apartment/Hospital Research http://highwayhypodermics.com/wp/travel-nursing-information/free-travel-nursing-forms/

Highway Hypodermics: Travel Company Referrals – Choosing a travel company can be very difficult with over 400 travel nursing companies competing for nurses. The following form can be used to send your information to those companies affiliated to this website. All that is required is a name and email address at the minimum: http://highwayhypodermics.com/wp/questionnaires/travel-company-referrals/

Facebook: Highway Hypodermics (the official FB page): Our Facebook site that keeps you up to date with new travel nursing news, special offers, and our job lists from our great sponsors! https://www.facebook.com/HighwayHypodermics/

Facebook: Travel Nursing Newbies: This is a group started by Kay (Epi) Slane and sponsored by Highway Hypodermics ®, LLC, for nurses who are wanting to jump into the big world of travel healthcare. This is a place that newbies can come and get their questions answered freely, truthfully, and honestly while reinforcing the idea of a great travel nurse. This group does include experienced recruiters and experienced traveling nurses that are willing to help out new traveling healthcare professionals. They promote flexibility, integrity, adaptability, professionalism, and dependability. https://www.facebook.com/groups/TravelNursingNewbies/

Facebook: Travel Nursing Newbie Recruiters: As important as it is for new traveling nurses to learn how to be a great travel nurse, I believe that it is equally important for a new recruiter to learn how to do things the right way the first time. I personally have gone to several travel companies and put on a training program titled "Got Nurses?" This group is an extension of that idea teaching recruiters what traveling nurses REALLY want in a company. https://www.facebook.com/groups/travelnursingnewbierecruiters/

Facebook: Highway Hypodermics RV Travelers: A group for traveling nurses, spouses, and allied healthcare professionals to come together and support each other while traveling across the United States in a recreational vehicle. There are members who have travel trailers, 5th wheels, Class C RVs and Class As. https://www.facebook.com/groups/HighwayHypodermicsRvTravelers/

Facebook: Homeschooling Rn Travel Nurses: A small group of traveling nurses and allied healthcare professionals that have decided to hit the road and homeschool their children. Even if you are only curious, come on over and join us! https://www.facebook.com/groups/HomeschoolingRnTravelNurses/

~*~

Travel Tax – Tax preparation for travel nurses and other traveling medical and mobile professionals. Having worked as a travel respiratory therapist for over three years, Joseph's background provides a superior understanding of tax issues for the mobile professional. New clients are always welcome and initial consultations are always free. www.traveltax.com

PAN Travelers – The Professional Association of Nurse Travelers serves as a comprehensive educational resource for Healthcare Travelers in the United States. Our larger vision is to improve the conditions for Healthcare Travelers, hospitals and patients. The Association identifies issues of concern to nurse travelers, researches solutions, and defines standards that foster safe, healthy, and humane work environments. www.pantravelers.org

Travelers Conference – The Traveler's Conference is an annual event that provides Traveling Healthcare Professionals an opportunity to network with other travelers and top industry insiders. You will earn CEU's for classes specific to the industry, and meet agency representatives in a relaxed, low-pressure setting. This event has grown into the largest gathering of healthcare travelers in the United States. For Travelers – By Travelers! www.travelersconference.com

Blue Pipes – Blue Pipes is a professional networking platform dedicated to healthcare professionals. Their mission is simple: provide healthcare professionals with unique career management tools to help them manage their careers more efficiently and successfully. www.bluepipes.com

Delphi Travel Nurses & Therapists Forum, TNT – A unique collection of medical professionals. They come to offer and find community support, answers to our questions and to meet fellow travelers. We are here to share our knowledge and to assist in learning the ins and outs of the exciting life of the traveler. They also have a sister site forums. delphiforums.com/tntrecruiting, that are an excellent way to find your next assignment. http://forums.delphiforums.com/travelnurses/

Travel Nursing Central – The Travel Nursing Central website provides a community or central meeting place for health professional travelers to connect as well as gather and provide useful information. http://www.travelnurslingcentral.com/

Biographies

Know More about Epstein, Joe, and Aaron!

Epstein LaRue (aka Kay Slane, RN)

The writing world calls her Epstein LaRue, but reality calls her "Kay." No matter what you know her by, she is a lady of many talents. She has been a nurse since 1992, a published author since 2001, and a traveling nurse since 2003.

In 2001 and 2003 Epstein started her writing career with fictional romance novels, "Love At First Type" and "Crazy Thoughts of Passion." While these publications did not flourish into great sales, it gave her the motivation and courage to continue her passion for writing.

When she started travel nursing in 2003 things weren't as easy to find on the Internet and there was only one book on travel nursing. Disgusted by this process, she started writing down everything that she had learned and after her first travel assignment, started the manuscript for "Highway Hypodermics: Your Road Map to Travel Nursing." In September of 2005, this book was recognized by USA Book News as one of the top finalist for professional book of the year.

"Highway Hypodermics: Travel Nursing 2007" was released by Star Publish, LLC. The previous 143-page non-fictional work grew to over 290 pages. This was the first version to reach number one in the Nursing Trend, Issues, and Roles category on Amazon.

"Highway Hypodermics: On the Road Again" was published in 2009 and was recognized by USA Book News as one of the winners for professional reference book of the year, while two other travel nursing books ranked as finalist.

"Highway Hypodermics: Travel Nursing 2012" was the first edition to be published as an ebook. This book catapulted to number one on Amazon's nursing issues, trends, and roles list and hasn't left the top 100 since publication.

"Highway Hypodermics: Travel Nursing 2015" was the cross over into the category Amazon category of eBook: Medical Reference and often found its home in the top 100, hanging out with other books that start with the names of Lippincott, Mosby, Tabers, Davis, and the American Heart Association.

She has been published in "Nursing 2004," was a regular columnist in Healthcare Traveler magazine, and has authored several articles in Electorophysical Lab Digest. In December 2005, she was also named as a Healthcare Traveler of the year, and in 2007, her travel nursing website was featured on the Dr. Phil show with Travel Nursing Across America (episodes 738).

In 2013 she completed her Graduate-Level Certificate in Nursing Management (CGM) and currently travels as a house supervisor.

For more information about Epstein the author, visit her website at: *www.epsteinlarue.com.*

Joseph Smith, RRT/EA/mTax

Joseph finished degrees in Accounting and Respiratory Therapy, and worked as a travel respiratory therapist before founding TravelTax and TravelTax Canada, a tax practice catering to the travel healthcare professional and mobile professionals in other staffing segments. TravelTax is well known in the healthcare staffing industry and serves a substantial client base of domestic and international mobile professionals, and their staffing agencies. His firm prepares US and Canadian returns and represents clients before the IRS, Canadian Revenue Agency and State Tax Agencies in audits, tax controversies and litigation support.

Joseph is a regular contributor to a number of staffing related publications/social media. He is the co-author of the 2015 edition of Highway Hypodermics, serves on the Tax Compliance Committee of the National Association of Travel Healthcare Organizations (NATHO), a regular speaker at the Healthcare Staffing Summit and teaches taxation at Northeast Community College. In addition to his undergraduate degrees, Joseph holds a MS in Taxation from Golden Gate University and has completed tax courses at Athabasca University in Canada.

For more information about travel taxes, visit his website at: www. traveltax.com.

Aaron Highfill, RN, CFRN, International Traveler

Aaron has been traveling in some capacity for most of his life. He realized early on that traveling is more fun when someone else is paying for it. His nursing career has taken him to approximately two dozen countries, six continents, two cruise ships, one civil war, and a viral pandemic. When not traveling for work as a Flight Nurse for AMR Air Ambulance, he's probably traveling for fun.

Come to The Travelers Conference each fall to meet the authors!

Look For Our Next Book!

Highway Hypodermics: Travel Nursing 2019

to be released fall 2018

CPSIA information can be obtained
at www.ICGtesting.com
Printed in the USA
LVOW03s0105171017
552623LV00002B/358/P

9 781935 188810